# Narratives in Psychiatry

# Narratives in Psychiatry

*Maurice Greenberg, Sukhwinder Singh Shergill,*
*George Szmukler and Digby Tantam*

*Foreword by Anthony W. Clare*

Jessica Kingsley Publishers
London and Philadelphia

First published in the United Kingdom in 2003
by Jessica Kingsley Publishers Ltd
116 Pentonville Road
London N1 9JB, England
and
325 Chestnut Street
Philadelphia, PA 19106, USA

*www.jkp.com*

Copyright © 2003 Maurice Greenberg, Sukhwinder Singh Shergill,
George Szmukler and Digby Tantam

**Library of Congress Cataloging in Publication Data**
A CIP catalog record for this book is available from the Library of Congress

**British Library Cataloguing in Publication Data**
A CIP catalogue record for this book is available from the British Library

ISBN 1 84310 109 2

Printed and Bound in Great Britain by
Athenaeum Press, Gateshead, Tyne and Wear

# Contents

# *Foreword*

At the beginning of the twenty-first century, medicine appears and indeed sees itself to be robustly scientific and objective. There has been a steady stream of remarkable developments in our understanding of the biological basis of disease. In particular there are exciting advances in our understanding of molecular genetics, in the application of brain imaging and in the development of more specific and better-targeted drugs. So triumphant has been this march that critics have begun to warn of the neglect of the art of medicine. The importance of the relationship between physician and patient, significant in every specialty but crucial to the practice of psychiatry, is threatened by an undue reliance on technology. The professional literature and the public media are full of anguished concern and intense criticism concerning what is seen to be an erosion of confidence in the modern doctor as a listener, a communicator and a healer. And all of this is occurring at a time when the scientific gains in terms of diagnosis and treatment have never been more impressive.

This book serves to remind us that in psychiatry the diagnosis, course, treatment and outcome of disorders rest heavily on the extraordinarily complex and sensitive relationship between doctor and patient. In psychiatry in particular, but in medicine too, the patient contains all that needs to be known concerning what is going wrong and what needs to be attended to. For over a century now we have become so reliant on and bedazzled by tools that reveal so much – x-rays, assays, tissue samples, laboratory tests, chromosomal analysis and so on – that the most fundamental source of information, the patient's own account, becomes relegated to a lesser significance. Yet it remains a cardinal truth of good medical practice that much time, effort, heartache and money are saved by paying the most careful, systematic and informed attention to what, why and how the patient is saying what the patient has to say.

But this book does more. One of the reasons why there is so much public concern regarding such varied issues as the misuse of medical power, informed consent, patient compliance, confidentiality, inappropriate doctor–patient relationships and medical litigation is because what doctors and patients say and do to each other is not taken as seriously as the readings from machines. As the emphasis has shifted from what the patient has to say to what laboratory and other tests have to tell us, so doctors and other health care professionals have devalued the importance and impact of the therapeutic relationship. Worse, what has happened is that illness becomes something separate from the remainder of life, an external phenomenon to be tamed and despatched without too much attention being paid to the human being who is trying to make sense of what is happening, to absorb the experience of being ill within the overall context of his or her life. Too often in the interests of science doctors appear to commandeer disease and to see it as an enemy to be destroyed, leaving the individual a passive spectator at the battle. This book, with its emphasis on narrative, meaning, the relationship between subjective experience and objective reality, reasserts the primary truth of medicine, namely that establishing the true picture of health and disease requires the active participation of the patient at every stage.

It is a supreme irony that the modern doctor is more at ease in the understanding and management of the whole plethora of human organs – heart, lungs, kidneys, liver, spleen, gut, even brain – than he is with the human person, more at ease relating to the machinery than the totality of life. Making sense of psychiatric symptoms demands a comprehensive, multifaceted approach but so too does making sense of all disease and disorder. The challenge facing those branches of medicine where technology and the scientific method have already made a dramatic contribution is the same as that which faces psychiatry where the application of technology still remains a matter more of potential than of actual value – namely how are we to avoid losing sight of the person in the midst of bleeping machines and flickering computer screens. It is to the credit of the authors of this book that they have so sensibly and lucidly provided an answer.

*Anthony W. Clare, Professor of Psychiatry,*
*St Patrick's Hospital, Dublin.*

# Introduction

## Changes in psychiatric practice

Psychiatric practice has changed out of all recognition since we wrote *Making Sense of Psychiatric Cases* (Greenberg, Szmukler and Tantam 1986), the first edition of this book. Community based services are the rule, and psychiatrists now work much more closely in multiprofessional teams, so that more of their energy and time is devoted to supporting colleagues and overseeing treatment. Sometimes different professional perspectives offer models of understanding and care that may appear to conflict with, and challenge, the concept of mental illness. Public accountability of services, frequently highlighted following a death or an enquiry, has resulted in a raft of new recommendations that focus on the importance of, among other things, communication and risk management. Protocols to achieve these recommendations have been introduced, and although many of them include criteria that have been borrowed from psychiatric practice, the centrality of the skills required to be a clinician is no longer emphasized.

Under these circumstances the medical tradition of taking a careful history, undertaking a detailed clinical examination and formulating a treatment plan may seem out-dated and irrelevant. Since the application of these clinical skills is time-consuming and requires attention, it is easy to understand why short cuts are sought. As a consequence, acquisition of these skills can become neglected; even the relevance of a psychiatrist to the proper functioning of a clinical team may be questioned. Some psychiatrists have reacted to this change by emphasizing the overarching importance of the 'medical model' to mental health care. Although this may be understandable, it can result in continuing disputes about who is in charge, with damaging effects on team functioning and patient care.

Given all these changes, is there still a need for a book that focuses on clinical skills in psychiatry; particularly one that places the psychiatrist at the centre of patient care, that emphasizes the importance of obtaining information in a thorough manner, and that explains how this information is put together in a way that furthers understanding and treatment? Is it appropriate that the Royal College of Psychiatrists, in its professional examinations, requires candidates to demonstrate their ability to practise these skills?

In our view effective psychiatric practice requires a complex range of skills, including all those outlined above. However, we argue that its foundation is the ability to understand in particular ways individuals who experience mental illness. In order to achieve this psychiatrists not only need to be able to make a diagnosis, but also to be aware of how the illness may have been caused, the way in which it may reflect the interaction between the individual and his or her environment, its likely course, and the most effective treatment interventions. In addition, they must also learn how to contribute this knowledge to the overall care of patients in a way that is useful within the context of rapidly changing services. Although there is no short cut to acquiring these clinical skills, we hope that our book will help illuminate their value.

## How to use this book

Although we have followed the same outline as the previous edition, we have made a number of changes that reflect changes in practice and diagnosis, or otherwise improve the book. The narratives are briefer, with less repetition. The diagnoses used generally refer to either ICD10 (1992) or DSMIV (1994) classifications. However, where these differ in any significant clinical respect, we include a description of this.

The narratives are based on real situations, because we believe that placing the reader in life-like clinical situations is one of the best ways to learn about clinical practice. Each chapter begins with the problem as it presented to the psychiatrist. It then unfolds with a step-by-step demonstration of how we use the assessment to proceed from a mass of information about the symptoms, personal circumstances, and wishes of the patient to a plan of treatment. We would encourage readers to approach this actively, by practising how they would use the available information to think about their own assessment. This process should become easier as further chapters are read, particularly if readers compare and contrast their own views with those of the authors.

The narratives cover a broad range of psychiatric disorder and, apart from the first two chapters, can be read in any order. The first chapter is new, and describes in detail the principles of taking a history and conducting an examination, and how these are put together in an assessment. This chapter is particularly aimed at students and trainees who have virtually no experience of talking to patients presenting with mental health problems. We hope that it also helps explain the process to those with no knowledge of medicine. The second chapter illustrates how these principles can begin to be applied to an individual, through selection and organization. Subsequent chapters use material that has already, to some extent, been organized and selected.

## Some theoretical considerations

Our approach means there is little space for detailed theoretical discussion. Nevertheless, we think that it would be helpful to list some important themes that underpin our clinical practice. We hope that the reader will be stimulated to consider them more deeply.

### Clinical judgment

With practice, a competent interviewer would find most of the narratives reasonably straightforward to obtain and easy to communicate to others. However, what is significant in a particular situation may depend less on what is actually said than other, more subtle aspects of communication. For example, how a remark is put, the context in which it is made, the point in the course of a history when it emerges and the accompanying tone of voice may significantly affect its meaning.

Since we have attempted to preserve these observations the reader may sometimes conclude that we have drawn inferences which go well beyond the data provided. Some clinical judgments will depend on experience gained from previous similar cases and, sometimes, on intuition. However, intuitive judgments are highly subjective and therefore need to be constantly tested by seeking further information through history taking or by direct observation.

### Selection and organization

The structure we follow has a long tradition in British psychiatry. However, the narrative framework will influence both the information we seek and the value we place upon it. This may therefore limit how we conceptualize an individual's problems and impede the development of an original approach that might prove even more valuable. Although we do not discount this possibility we have found that the traditional assessment does allow considerable flexibility. Many models of mental illness can be subsumed and placed side by side within its framework; biological, psychodynamic, behavioural, family and social. Often this can be done without serious contradictions emerging, because some problems are better illuminated by adopting one view while others are better illuminated using another. When contradictions do arise, points of incompatibility are exposed and the evidence for the particular case can be marshalled to help us decide which approach is most helpful. Factors operate at a variety of conceptual levels in the clinical assessment, from the cultural to the biochemical, and can be integrated in a manner that is difficult to achieve in formal terms.

### The particular and the general

In every narrative the reader will become aware of our attention to two elements. We have sought to identify both the features that each individual has in common with others suffering from similar problems and those that are unique. The clinician needs to be mindful of both. Commonalities provide a link with a body of useful knowledge, empirically derived, concerning such matters as the general implications of a particular diagnosis or the likelihood that a particular treatment will be effective. However, the expression of a mental illness is also the product of an individual's unique circumstances, personality and past experiences. Our ability to establish rapport, or a working relationship, will be influenced by our understanding of how individuals see the world, their dispositions and their interests. We need to understand their 'language'. Throughout the assessment, the general and the particular stand side by side, each placing the other in perspective.

### Types of 'understanding'

We have employed a number of types, or levels, of 'understanding'. These go beyond the different 'models' of mental illness already mentioned. We attempt to build up a picture of how someone's problems have evolved by paying attention to their previous experiences, their vulnerabilities and resources and their current life circumstances. These features are particular to the individual and the processes involved cannot be expressed in terms of general laws. However, this enables a sequence of experiences to be comprehensible to the interviewer, who then understands how particular phenomena have arisen in an emphatic manner. This type of understanding (Jasper's *verstehen,* see Jaspers *et al.* 1988 for further explanation) is an everyday, practical one and depends on the interviewer's ability to see the imprint of a coherent individual consciousness or character in the individual's experiences and behaviour. However, it should also become apparent that in many instances this kind of understanding is insufficient to take us to the core of the morbid experiences to which our patients have been subject. A limit is reached beyond which the patient's experience and behaviour cannot be made sense of in this way. We might understand, for example, why someone has become distressed given their personality and life situation, but we cannot understand in the same sense why their illness has taken the form of a depressive psychosis rather than an anxiety state, or anorexia nervosa rather than an obsessive-compulsive neurosis. At this point we seek after a different kind of 'understanding' based on 'explanations'. Mental illnesses take the form of discontinuities in an individual's narrative that can be understood as catastrophes with a cause.

In contrast to emphatic 'understanding', 'causal explanations' are stated in scientific terms and are believed to follow general laws like those characterizing the natural sciences. They deal with factors, generally biological ones, operating at an extra-conscious level that can be studied using experimental methods. Their status as knowledge is different from that achieved through emphatic understanding.

The assessment, as presented in this book, heeds both 'understanding', which is underpinned by 'reasons' and 'explanation', underpinned by 'causes', and serves to define the relationships between them. Both are necessary for a full account of the development of an individual's illness.

## Eclecticism in treatment

The treatment offered arises out of the diagnostic and aetiological parts of the assessment. As clinicians, we are aware that our understanding of the patient cannot rest at an academic level, but must also lead to therapeutic implications. It could be argued that the major purpose of the formulation is a practical one; it enables us to offer help. Since the diagnosis and aetiology are usually multidimensional, so are the therapeutic options that develop from them. For example, a biological component may require medication and a psychological component may lead to the mobilization of social supports. Although one treatment modality may be particularly relevant, a single approach is generally insufficient, and the sequencing of treatment is often important. For example, medication may need to be given before someone can become accessible to psychotherapeutic help. The assessment acts as a corrective to the slavish adherence to a single kind of treatment.

We hope the reader will find our approach persuasive not only for theoretical and practical reasons, but also because it demonstrates that an assessment can be more than a dry-as-dust examination exercise. We will have been successful if readers are able to imagine themselves responsible for each individual described. Since psychiatry is not yet a very exact science we would expect there to be disagreement about the management we have described. Whether this happens or not, we shall be satisfied if readers are stimulated to be more precise or more comprehensive in their own assessments, especially if they find, as we do, that the clinical experience gained from each assessment hones up a technical skill that can subsequently be exercised with greater economy of effort and to a higher standard.

## References

American Psychiatric Association (1994) *Diagnostic and Statistical Manual of Mental Disorders, Fourth Edition. (DSM-IV)*. Washington, DC: APA.

Greenberg, M., Szmukler, G. and Tantam, D. (1986) *Making Sense of Psychiatric Cases.* Oxford: Oxford University Press.

World Health Organisation (1992) *The ICD-10 Classification of Mental and Behavioural Disorders.* Geneva: WHO.

# Chapter 1

# Information Gathering

Psychiatry is unusual in the degree to which it relies on clinical skills. This chapter describes a framework that is intended to help the student in the acquisition and practice of these skills. It is divided into three sections; the psychiatric interview, examination of the mental state, and the psychiatric assessment. These three aspects of management are, in practice, closely linked, and they have only been separated for the sake of clarity and convenience.

## General principles

The psychiatric interview has the potential to be both therapeutic and educational. Its impact will depend upon the manner in which it is conducted, since developing a satisfactory therapeutic alliance will only improve the quality of any information that is obtained. Having a clear and comprehensible framework within which to collect information facilitates interviewing. The one provided here is based upon the principle that a detailed account of an individual's psychiatric problem will be illuminated by an understanding of that person's development, which includes personal, social and biological dimensions.

An initial psychiatric interview takes about an hour to complete. It is important to undertake this without interruption, and it is useful to leave some time at the end, so that the information that has been obtained can be organized.

This information is inevitably highly personal, and the manner in which the interview is conducted needs to convey respect, seriousness, sensitivity and human compassion. Although this might mean that some lines of enquiry should be delayed until a later occasion, it is important to cover the major areas outlined below, but at the same time to show tact when approaching difficult issues.

It is unlikely that people undergoing their first psychiatric interview will ever have been offered so much uninterrupted time to talk about themselves and their problems. The impact of this, and the inevitable hope that they will be helped, will be to encourage powerful expectations of the interviewer. This can be useful, because it is likely to facilitate cooperation, which in turn is likely to further treatment. However, it can be difficult if they are left feeling 'high and dry' afterwards. A joint appraisal towards the end of the interview can help minimize this by conveying the sense that their opinions will be treated with respect. It is also reassuring if the psychiatrist can offer an explanation of how he or she makes sense of the problems that have emerged and what can be done about them. This is not always easy – because the problem is too complicated for a simple explanation, because the interviewer has not obtained sufficient information to have got to the bottom of it, or from a combination of these factors. In such circumstances, it can be helpful to acknowledge that it is unrealistic to be able to offer a simple explanation after only one meeting.

Finally, the interviewer should always consider whether a physical examination is indicated. This is a routine part of a psychiatric inpatient assessment, and may reveal some previously unexpected disorder that is relevant to the presenting problem. It needs to be undertaken if there is any suspicion that such a disorder exists.

## The setting

Psychiatric interviews can take place in many different settings, such as a general hospital ward, a casualty department, an individual's home, or a prison. This is likely to affect the question the psychiatrist needs to answer. For example, should someone who has taken an overdose be admitted to hospital, or does someone arrested for a criminal offence suffer from a mental illness which might have affected his or her responsibility? The approach described here is likely to be particularly constrained by the amount of time available for the interview, as well as by the situation. If time is limited it will be necessary to make important decisions first, and to provide time for a more detailed assessment later. This will allow an opportunity to reflect, to discuss any problems with colleagues, and to see the person again in another setting.

Although it is customary for the 'patient' to be interviewed first, this is not inevitable, and some psychiatrists, particularly those used to working with families or couples, will see the relevant parties together from the outset. It is also likely that psychiatrists, whatever their approach, will want to interview other family members or friends, in order to substantiate or clarify details that are relevant to reaching a diagnosis and organizing management.

The most difficult decisions tend to be about the need for urgent admission, such as when someone who has taken an overdose is being examined in the casualty department. At such times the duty psychiatrist may feel torn between the conflicting demands from the casualty department to 'move the patient', and from the psychiatric ward to protect beds for people who are extremely ill. The patient's view and that of the patient's family may also be in conflict about admission. Under these circumstances psychiatrists must insist on completing as detailed an examination as they consider necessary in order to make the appropriate decision.

## The psychiatric interview

### The presenting complaint

The interview usually begins by asking about the current problem, which needs to be described as clearly as possible, using the patient's own words. This can be facilitated by getting into the habit of writing down exactly what the patient says, and how the conversation develops. For example, patients may begin by saying that they feel 'depressed'. Sometimes 'depressed' may have a personal meaning, such as a voice saying 'what a horrible person I am', and not an alteration in mood or self-esteem. In these circumstances a serious error can arise if this is not established at the outset. However, even when patients are referring to their mood and suffering from a depressive illness, to say that the presenting problem is depression tells us next to nothing about what is going on. Depression affects different people in different ways. The psychiatrist needs to know how severe it is, what are its effects, what seems to bring it on and how long it has being going on. In depression, specific changes may occur in sleeping or eating habits as well as in other areas of biological functioning; if such symptoms are not volunteered spontaneously they must be asked about directly.

This illustrates further useful principles for conducting an interview:

- Ensure, as far as possible, that you understand what patients mean.

- Begin with open-ended questions such as 'Can you tell me about your problem?' and gradually introduce more direction, 'What do you mean by depression?', before bringing in clear-cut choices or using closed questions, 'Has your depression affected your appetite?'

Using an open-ended approach and recording exactly what is said will produce an account that is less contaminated by the psychiatrist's preconceptions. However, this can be a lengthy procedure and it is often necessary to use direction and shorthand in one area of an examination in order to concentrate on particular issues in another. Knowing when to use a more directive approach is a skill acquired through experience and intuition, and requires considerable practice in talking and listening to patients.

By using this process of active and interested enquiry the psychiatrist should be in a position to answer the following questions about the presenting problem:

- What is its nature?

- How severe is it?

- How did it start (suddenly, or gradually, or in relation to any particular event)?

- When did it start?
- How has it affected the individual's level of functioning?
- Is there anything that aggravates or alleviates it?
- Has it ever happened before?

Seeking answers to these questions in a respectful and sensitive way should enable patients to communicate something of their concerns. They are likely to experience some relief and also be forthcoming about themselves. At this stage it is appropriate to turn to the biographical enquiry.

## Family history

The family history begins with an account of parents and siblings which, when appropriate, can be extended to include other family members. The following information about family members should be obtained: their age, employment, health (including mental health) and a general appraisal of their personalities and relationships. The psychiatrist is likely to get some idea of the general atmosphere of the family – such as whether it was warm, close-knit and caring, or cold, distant and unemotional. An impression is also likely to be gained of which relationships were particularly important, and whether they have been sustained. These aspects should be further clarified, so that the interviewer develops a feeling for what it may have been like to be a member of this family.

## Personal history

The personal history follows the family history, because individual development emerges from within the framework of the nuclear family. Some details of very early development should now be asked about. These include whether the patient was premature, breast-fed, or suffered any separation from his or her parents. Such events may have a profound effect upon the initial 'bonding' process between a mother and her infant, which can influence later relationships. Although most people can remember their childhood it is unusual for them to be completely honest about this with a stranger, particularly if it arouses unpleasant feelings. They are also likely to consider their childhood 'normal' since they have nothing to compare it with. A result of this is that early childhood and development are frequently described as 'normal' even when there have been significant conflicts and separations. More realistic descriptions are only likely to be provided when the psychiatrist has established confidence and is sensitive to subtle clues that can be followed up tactfully.

It is important to enquire into both the relationships that existed within the family and its socio-cultural context. Was it representative of any particular group and did this reflect the local neighbourhood? For example, a professional, two-parent family living in a middle-class neighbourhood will provide a very different set of experiences to that of a single-parent family living in a deprived inner-city area.

Having explored home life and social context, the next step is to discover how the patient related to people outside the family. This begins with an account of early friendships and how the patient coped with entering school. Whether patients enjoyed meeting other people, were popular, and engaged in social activities and sport, are all as important as whether they were academically successful. This information will help build up a picture of the patient's personality – outgoing or isolated, easy-going or argumentative, and so on. It will also provide a 'narrative' aspect to the development so the interviewer will get a 'feel' for a sense of continuity. The history will either unfold coherently, with each succeeding stage fitting in with the previous information, or surprises may occur, such as when an intelligent person does unexpectedly badly in an examination. Explanations for such discontinuities in the narrative are likely to provide further understanding.

An account of the patient's academic achievement will give a general idea of intellectual ability, and how he or she got on with teachers provides an early example of relationships with people in authority outside the home. Whether the individual was a prefect or had a reputation as a troublemaker would also be relevant to this aspect.

This is followed by a history of further education and will lead into employment history. It remains important to know about the relationships that developed during these periods of time. It is also necessary to know the patient's pattern of work. Were there long periods of unemployment, and if so, why? Were there numerous jobs, only lasting for a brief period of time, or was there satisfactory career progress, with promotions? If retired, it would be necessary to know how well this had been planned, and whether it had been experienced as an enjoyable change.

By the time this information has been gathered an increasingly clear picture of the patient should be emerging. Most patients will probably feel that the psychiatrist has begun to know them pretty well and will therefore be less embarrassed about discussing their psychosexual history. For a woman this will involve an account of her menarche and menopause (if relevant) and any associated emotional complications. It is also important to know whether she has had any pregnancies, miscarriages or terminations, and how she reacted to these. For both men and women it will include a history of important emotional and sexual relationships, including a description of current relationships. This will include an assessment of how satisfactory the patient finds his or her partner, both emotionally as well as sexually. An effective way of gauging the degree of sexual satisfaction is to ask how frequently they have sexual intercourse, and whether this has recently changed. If the patient is not in a relationship similar questions can be asked about masturbation.

Most people will have suffered a significant loss or separation at some time during their lives, and it is always necessary to discover how they coped with this experience, including whether they were able to mobilize any support from friends and family to help them.

The history will have now reached the stage at which the present problem began to develop. It should be possible to see whether this was preceded by any significant life changes, which might have been minimized earlier in the interview, such as the loss of a job or the end of a relationship.

There are two other aspects of the history that should always be enquired into if they have not yet emerged. The first is whether there has been any abuse of alcohol or other drugs. This requires asking 'what' and 'how much', not just 'whether' the patient drinks. The second is whether there has been evidence of any antisocial behaviour or contact with the law. The details of any act of violence need to be known, including its severity, the nature of any precipitants, whether weapons were used, and the consequences. Any suspicious clues should result in a detailed history of both these areas.

## Past medical history

It is always necessary to obtain a detailed account of any illness that has required medical treatment. This should include not only the diagnosis, when it occurred and how it was treated, but also the symptoms and manifestations and whether it resulted in any long-term difficulties. A list of any medication prescribed currently or within the previous few months should always be included.

## Past psychiatric history

Similar principles apply to those outlined in the previous section. However, it is generally useful to think in broader terms than whether someone has simply been treated in the past by their family doctor, or by a psychiatrist. Many people experience minor psychiatric disturbances that may neither be brought to their doctor's attention, nor even be recognized. It is therefore sensible to ask whether there have been experiences similar to the present ones or any subjectively marked alterations in mood. If so, it will then be necessary to find out the circumstances in which these occurred. The personal history may have revealed clues to such events. For example, 'considerable apprehension' about attending school might, on more detailed questioning, reveal a clear description of school phobia and school refusal.

## Previous personality

A picture should now have begun to emerge of the sort of person the patient was before his or her problem developed. We are as interested in patients' strengths as we are in their weaknesses and should therefore always note these, including any outstanding characteristic, such as being particularly isolated, gregarious, passive, or argumentative. This section should also include aspects that highlight the current problem. For example, if patients are depressed it would be important to know whether they were usually the 'life and soul' of the party or had always tended to be miserable. The way they coped with previous adversity, such as examination failures, may also offer insight into their personality.

Finally, we are particularly interested in the relationships patients have developed. Do they make friends easily, and do they keep them? Are their relationships stereotyped, following a predictable pattern, or do they have a wide range of friends, some of whom they have maintained over a long period of time?

This sort of information is best derived indirectly, rather than by asking, 'What sort of person do you think you are?' It can be inferred from the personal history, but should also be supplemented and corroborated by an independent informant. Furthermore, during the interview the psychiatrist may begin to experience a 'feel' for the relationship that is developing with the patient.

## Examination of the mental state

The different systems, or sub-divisions, of the mental state used in this book follow those described in most textbooks of undergraduate and postgraduate psychiatry.

They are as follows:

- Appearance and general behaviour
- Speech
- Mood
- Thought content
- Abnormal beliefs and interpretations of events
- Abnormal experiences (related to environment, body or self)
- The cognitive state
- Self-appraisal.

The changes that can occur within the mental state as a result of specific psychiatric disorders are well described in a number of psychiatric textbooks (see Further Reading, p.36). Here we concentrate upon general principles and use examples to illustrate them.

The first of these principles applies to the recording of the mental state which, like the history, needs to make use of the individual's own words as far as possible. The mental state is what the patient says, thinks, or does and the way in which this comes across. The second principle is that it is important to try to organize the mental state within the different systems described. This may appear complicated and time-consuming to begin with, particularly as there is some degree of arbitrariness about the distinctions, but it will help improve students' clinical skill by encouraging them to be specific in their psychiatric descriptions. In practice it is more realistic if the account is recorded verbatim and is organized after the interview has been completed. However, particularly when learning, it is easy to forget some areas of the mental state. At this stage it is therefore helpful to have a checklist of questions in mind. Finally, as will be described in the section on assessment, not all the necessary information will be obtained at one sitting. Further interviews are nearly always necessary in order to fill in gaps in the information, or to clarify certain details. Often, these will involve interviews with other informants, such as relatives or friends.

APPEARANCE AND GENERAL BEHAVIOUR

The description of appearance and behaviour should be life-like and clearly convey any notable abnormality. Although it is impossible to list every possible aspect, it will often begin with a description of the way the patient is dressed, which will include what they are wearing as well as whether it is tidy, clean, shabby, or obviously inappropriate. Their demeanour should also be recorded. This includes whether they look sad or happy, retain a fixed posture or move around freely and in a relaxed fashion, appear tense and agitated or relaxed, seem to concentrate on the interview or to be easily distractible, and whether their overall behaviour seems to be consistent with what they are talking about as well as appropriate to the context of the examination. Any obvious facial grimaces or abnormal body movements should be described in this section. Although a description of the quality of eye contact with the interviewer can provide a useful index of the interaction, cultural factors always need to be considered before drawing inferences. An example of this is 'good eye contact'. In Western culture, maintaining a direct gaze is seen as a sign of autonomy and respect, whereas in Indian culture it signals disrespect if someone looks directly at a 'more senior' person.

Sometimes, even when patients cannot, or will not, talk about themselves, their behaviour may suggest that they are subject to psychotic experiences. Under these circumstances they may appear to be listening to another person talking, they may stare into space or gesticulate, and their facial expression may suggest that they are involved in a heated discussion.

There are a number of reasons why patients may not speak during an interview. They may have a depressive stupor, a brain lesion, or wilfully choose to remain mute. Examination of the mental state can help to distinguish between the possible causes and requires a detailed description of the appearance and behaviour. For example, if they are depressed they are likely to look miserable and move very slowly, if they have elective mutism they are less likely to sustain a fixed alteration of mood and movement, and if they have a brain lesion they are more likely to exhibit neurological signs.

SPEECH

This section is for what is called the form, rather than the content, of speech: how things are said, not what is said. The rate, fluency and coherence of speech should all be described, as well as whether it is spontaneous, relevant to the topic being discussed and maintains the point.

Formal disorders of thought should be described here. This confusing term can refer to the seemingly disconnected thought processes, thought block and neologisms of schizophrenia; or to the flight of ideas found in mania; or to the perseveration, echolalia and incoherence that may occur in dementing disorders. Since the distinction between these is vital in helping to establish a diagnosis, an accurate and detailed verbatim record should always be used as an illustration.

MOOD

The account of how patients describe their feelings needs to be embellished with observations of features such as their facial expression and posture, and also how they describe events in their lives. Sometimes there may be subtle clues. They may seem to skirt away from a subject that appears to be painful, or appear to be making an effort to hide sadness by presenting themselves as excessively cheerful. In practice, interviewers are generally more aware of attempts to mask sad feelings than of a mild elevation in mood, which is frequently overlooked.

The quality of the emotional state can be described in many different terms, such as whether someone is happy, sad, anxious, irritable, suspicious, frightened, or perplexed. It should also be noted whether the mood is fixed or fluctuates during the interview. If it varies, does this appear to be in response to what is being discussed and is it appropriate? Most people can become heated when they discuss something that they care about, such as politics or sport. It is also appropriate to become upset and to cry when talking about a lost relative whom one loved. However, it is unusual to sustain such extreme moods regardless of the topic of conversation. It is also inappropriate to laugh uproariously when discussing a sad loss, or to cry desperately when recounting a happy experience. The mood is described as 'flat' if there is reduced responsiveness associated with an absence of feeling. This contrasts with a 'labile' mood and is different in quality to a 'fixed' mood, which can be very intense, as may occur in severe depression.

In certain situations patients may seem to be denying their true feelings. However, 'denial' implies a conscious or unconscious activity, and interviewers should ensure that they are not simply attributing what they believe to be the hidden emotional response. One important clue to this may be if the individual categorically states that they do not have a particular feeling without having been asked about it. However, if it is unclear it is better to stick to a simple description of what the patient does, or does not, feel.

Finally, particularly if patients are depressed or irritable, it is essential to ask whether they have ever thought of harming themselves. Many students are worried about asking this question because they think they may put the idea into someone's mind. In practice, however, patients are far more likely to feel relief at sharing the burden of such thoughts with someone who is not shocked by them, and will often go on to describe how ashamed and isolated they have felt about them. In order to find this out in as helpful a way as possible, both the timing and the manner in which the question is put are important. The style should be sympathetic and non-judgmental. The question should follow from what is being discussed, rather than being tacked on because it needs to be asked. For example, when patients talk about something that has upset them, and are describing how miserable they feel, it makes sense to say something like, 'Did it ever get so bad that you felt like harming yourself?' or 'Have you felt that it was difficult to go on?' If the answer is 'Yes' then it will be necessary to explore this further by asking whether they have made any plans to harm themselves, what they are, how far they have proceeded, and whether they have made any attempts on other occasions. All of these factors give some indication of the severity of suicidal risk.

THOUGHT CONTENT

This should summarize patients' main thoughts and worries. Particular attention should be paid to morbid thoughts, which seem to be obviously unusual, exaggerated, or distressing, and with which they seem to be preoccupied. Although these will often become apparent spontaneously, it is always appropriate to ask what they think are their main problems.

There are many different ways of categorizing thoughts. It is therefore best to describe them briefly, using the individual's own language, and then to illustrate their most notable characteristic. Are they mainly about the patient him or herself or about others; about the present, future or past; about real or imaginary events; are they violent or bland? If the thoughts seem quite ordinary and appropriate to the situation, this should be stated.

Often, it is their thoughts that patients complain about. In these circumstances their nature, and in what way they have caused problems, should be clarified. If patients are very anxious, for example, they will frequently describe the same worries as 'going around and around my mind' and say that they prevent them from falling asleep or from concentrating on their work.

Abnormal thoughts should be described here. These include phobias, which are intense fears of a particular object or situation, resulting in considerable anxiety and a desire to avoid that object or situation. Sometimes a phobia will be experienced as irrational, but this is not always so. A fairly common example of this is a spider-phobia. Agoraphobia, literally a fear of open spaces, is used to describe a generalized phobic state, or 'free-floating anxiety'.

Obsessional ruminations are persistently recurring thoughts that are experienced as unpleasant, that are often, but not always, perceived as ridiculous, and that people make efforts to eradicate. An example of this might be when a very devout person becomes bothered by a blasphemous thought, such as 'bugger the Church'. Unlike hallucinations (see below) the person is in no doubt that the thought emanates from his or her own mind, but is at a loss to explain it.

A compulsion is an irresistible urge to repeat an action, even though the purpose is seen as irrational. It is the behavioural equivalent of an obsession, and frequently arises as a consequence of one. For example, it may be appropriate to check the locks once or twice when going out, particularly if there has been a spate of burglaries. However, it becomes a compulsion when it has to be repeated many times, even though one knows that all the doors are locked. A variation of this is a ritual, which is a complicated series of actions repeated whenever the same task is performed. Sometimes a ritual is appropriate, such as when an electrician checks that the electricity is off before servicing a television. It becomes pathological when it takes up excessive time and is performed unnecessarily: for example, when a person can only wash if towels are folded in a particular fashion, if the soap is on the correct side of the sink, if the basin is filled to the correct level, if all these separate activities have to be carried out in the same order, and if even a minor change occurs in this pattern the person then has to return to the beginning and start all over again.

ABNORMAL BELIEFS AND INTERPRETATIONS OF EVENTS

An individual's beliefs, and his or her explanation for what is happening, will generally become apparent while the history is unfolding. However, paranoid, secretive, or sensitive people may keep such ideas hidden, particularly if they are aware that they may become incorporated into a diagnosis. Under these circumstances, if the psychiatrist is suspicious, it may be necessary to ask directly about 'feeling controlled' or 'people talking about you'.

Any abnormal beliefs should first be described in the individual's own words. They then need to be clarified so that the psychiatrist understands, for example, what 'something strange going on' means. The psychiatrist also needs to know how firmly the beliefs are held, and the extent to which they are incorporated into a view of the world. Testing this aspect of belief systems can be difficult, because it involves challenging something that is central to a patient's world. However, it is surprising how often people with severely disordered thoughts, which permeate their lives, will accept with equanimity that other people do not agree with them. This is particularly true if the interviewer is open about this and makes it clear that the patient's integrity is not being challenged. Although the particular style will vary according to the situation, one way of approaching this issue is to say something like: 'Do you think everyone sees it like this?'

The fact that someone tenaciously holds on to a belief that is commonly accepted as abnormal is not necessarily a manifestation of psychiatric illness. Many people have eccentric ideas that may not be acceptable to others. An example of this is someone who fervently believes that the earth is flat and has joined the 'flat earth society'. This applies even when it does not appear to be so acceptable, as when someone believes in witchcraft, joins a witches' coven and practises satanic rites. Although this may not be normal behaviour for the population as a whole, it is normal in our society for groups to exist that follow their own, separate rules, which are consistent with their own sub-culture.

Frequently an explanation can be found for people holding such beliefs, without invoking a morbid psychiatric process; for example, they may come from a family that has always shown an interest in similar activities. The psychiatric term for such a belief is an 'over-valued idea', and this needs to be distinguished from a delusion, which does signal the presence of a serious psychiatric illness. A delusion is an abnormal belief which is held with unshakeable intensity and which is inexplicable solely in terms of the person's upbringing, culture and personality. The difference between an over-valued idea and a delusion may not always be clear-cut. However, they can generally be distinguished by establishing how long the belief has been held, how it developed, how consistent it is with the individual's general attitudes and whether there is any other evidence of a morbid psychological process. Delusions are not life-long beliefs (certainly so far as the quality with which they are professed is concerned). They tend to develop out of the blue (in schizophrenia) or out of a severely altered mood (in affective disorders) and they cannot be understood solely in terms of personality and circumstances, without invoking extraordinary explanations. They may also occur in organic brain syndromes, when there will be other evidence of the underlying disorder. (See 'The cognitive state', below.)

Delusions may be distinguished by their particular qualities. They should therefore be described in detail, which includes the quality with which they are held. Some psychiatrists distinguish between 'primary' and 'secondary' delusions, meaning that they have arisen out of a disturbance of belief, or an alteration of mood, respectively. In practice this is another way of saying 'schizophrenic' or 'affective' and is an attempt to rate their understandability. Such distinctions can be confusing and it is better to simply state that a delusion is held and to describe it clearly. Any possible causes should be discussed in the assessment. A person may also misinterpret events going on around them. They may believe that people talking together in a public house are talking about them, and that this has been confirmed when one of them smiles in their direction. This experience is called an 'idea of reference', and may or may not be associated with the presence of delusions.

ABNORMAL EXPERIENCES (RELATED TO ENVIRONMENT, BODY OR SELF)

In this section it is important to distinguish between 'hallucinations', which are sensory experiences occurring in the absence of external stimulation, and 'illusions', which are misinterpretations of sensory stimulations. Either of these can be experienced through any of the sensory modalities. Illusions are part of normal experience, such as when shadows in a poorly lit street may appear to be lurking people (particularly when one is feeling somewhat anxious). Hallucinations generally reflect a morbid change, although they do occur in normal situations. For example, after his wife's death a man may hear her voice calling him, or feel her lying in bed next to him. Two other types of 'normal' hallucination occur when someone is just waking, or just falling asleep, called hypnopompic and hypnogogic, respectively.

This section should also contain a description of any episodes of 'derealization' (the experience that things around are not real) or of 'depersonalization' (when the individual feels unreal). The latter is often described as 'feeling as if I was standing outside myself, looking on'. The degree of fixity of the experience should always be tested, and a distinction drawn between those experiences that are certain and those that are not. Patients can often distinguish between these and describe the latter as 'as if' experiences.

The experience that an external agency is interfering with thoughts and stopping them is called 'thought block'. Sometimes this distressing symptom will be described clearly, but often it can only be inferred from the fact that the flow of speech is interrupted with silences. It is pathognomic of schizophrenia, and needs to be distinguished from a similar experience that commonly occurs in severe anxiety, when the individual may say, 'It was *as if* the thoughts had been taken out of my head.'

As has already been emphasized in each section, it is insufficient to state that the patient has had an hallucination; the details need to be described. These include its content, where it was felt to come from, how frequently it was experienced, and whether there was anything that clearly provoked or stopped it.

## THE COGNITIVE STATE

This part of the examination covers the patient's orientation, attention and concentration, and memory. It also includes an assessment of their intelligence.

The cognitive state is likely to be normal in the majority of presentations to an adult psychiatrist, and can be judged as such without resorting to particular tests. In general, abnormalities will become apparent through the history and how it is presented. For example, a patient may complain of a failing memory, repeat themselves, and persist in giving obviously inaccurate information. In such circumstances a complete cognitive assessment should be undertaken. However, practically every psychiatrist will remember one occasion when a cognitive deficit was missed, because it was not specifically looked for, and it is always worthwhile making a general assessment. The Mini Mental State Examination is a clinically useful brief screening instrument, and a more detailed and thorough examination will need to be performed when there is any suspicion of cognitive deficit.

- *Orientation*: This should be tested in relation to the individual (can they remember their name), in space (do they know where they are) and in time (do they know the time).

- *Attention and concentration*: The ability of patients to give a coherent, lucid, continuous account of themselves will generally demonstrate any problems in this area. This is particularly so if they are also able to respond appropriately to the interviewer's questions, without seeming to lose their way. A simple way of testing this is to ask them to continue subtracting 7s from 100, to time this, and note any mistakes.

- *Memory*: This should manifest itself in the history. If a memory defect is suspected it should be noted whether it is global or selective. Most dementing illnesses result in changes in recent memory to begin with, and sometimes 'confabulation', when gaps in memory are filled with false information.

- *Intelligence*: An overall evaluation of intelligence can be made on the account of the patient's education, interests and achievements. It is always important to note inconsistencies between what is observed during the examination, and what would be expected from the history. For example, a small deterioration in intellectual functioning is likely to affect a manual worker in different ways to a professor of physics, both in the impact it would have on his or her general level of functioning, as well as the subtlety of change that might manifest itself during a psychiatric interview.

A thorough and detailed cognitive assessment and the use of specific intelligence tests are both specialized tasks, covered in the textbooks.

SELF-APPRAISAL

This section provides an opportunity for patients to describe what they think is wrong with them and their attitude towards this. Although this may well have been covered in previous sections, it is useful to bring together the relevant information here, because it draws attention to factors that will influence the eventual management. For example, if they recognize that their problem is psychological rather than physical, and can acknowledge the importance of stressful experience in its development, it suggests that they are 'psychologically minded' and able to make use of psychotherapy. On the other hand, if they are depressed, and insist that their problem is due to physical changes and will not respond favourably to any treatment, they are likely to need physical treatment.

Sometimes a decision has to be made about the extent to which an illness has interfered with a patient's ability to make informed choices about his or her own welfare. This can be a complicated problem and its resolution will depend partly upon the acceptability of the patient's own explanation, the patient's preferred treatment option and attitude to alternatives.

THE ASSESSMENT

When the examination has been completed, the information obtained needs to be selected and organized in order to develop an effective management plan. The assessment is the application of relevant psychiatric knowledge to what has been discovered. Learning to write a psychiatric assessment should help interviewers structure their thoughts in a psychiatric way, without losing sight of the importance of the individual. After a brief description of the salient features of the history and examination, the assessment is discussed under the following headings: Diagnosis; Aetiology; Further information; Management; Prognosis.

These categories will occasionally be refined in the light of additional information. We have also included postscripts, because not every situation will have been 'closed'. Finally, the stories described here reflect the real world, in that errors and misjudgments are included. Readers are therefore invited to consider how they might have reached different conclusions or made different judgments. We hope that this will encourage them to become active participants in thinking about people with psychiatric disorders.

## Further Reading

### General Textbooks

Gelder, M., Lopez-Ibor, J.J. and Andreasen, N. (Eds) (2000) *New Oxford Textbook of Psychiatry*. Oxford: Oxford University Press.

Goldberg, D. and Murray, R (eds) (2002) *Maudsley Handbook of Practical Psychiatry*. Oxford: Oxford University Press.

Johnstone, E.C., Freeman, C.P.L. And Zealley, A.K. (Eds) (1998) *Companion to Psychiatric Studies*. Edinburgh: Churchill Livingstone.

Murray, R., Hill, P. and McGuffin, P (eds) (1997) *The Essentials of Postgraduate Psychiatry*. Cambridge: Cambridge University Press.

### Psychopathology

Bolton, D. And Hill, J. (1996) *Mind, Meaning and Mental Disorder*. Oxford: Oxford University Press.

Jaspers, K. (1998) *General Psychopathology Vol. 1&2*. Baltimore: The Johns Hopkins University Press.

Sims, A (1995) *Symptoms in the Mind*. Ontario: Saunders.

*Chapter 2*

# Developing a Narrative
## Mr Daniels

### Presenting complaint

The staff of a local day centre contacted the hospital to ask for help. Mr Daniels, a 17-year-old Guyanese-born man who had been attending the day centre regularly for some time, had recently begun to behave strangely, and they felt that they could no longer cope with him. The last straw was when he came into a staff meeting, insisting that he was a member of staff, and spent the meeting kneeling in a position of prayer, making bellowing noises.

Further questioning over the telephone elicited the information that he had been odd for several days, and that he had stated on different occasions that he was dead and that half his brain was linked to the moon. He lived in his own flat with an older brother. It was thought that he would probably need admission, and it was suggested that he be brought immediately to the hospital.

When he arrived he sat down in a cubicle within the Accident and Emergency Department, but kept his eyes closed and either refused to answer questions, or shouted 'No!' to them. He did however respond physically to simple requests and it was possible to make a superficial physical examination, which showed an axillary temperature of 38.5°C and a radial pulse rate of 120. He seemed hostile and suspicious, but not depressed.

At this point, Mr Daniel's mother, who worked nearby, arrived. She said that Mr Daniels appeared well until two weeks before, when he visited and seemed rather restless. A week before, on another visit, he had sworn at her, 'a sure sign of illness' according to his mother, and tried to set fire to a book on the kitchen stove, saying, 'After this I'll be all right because I'll be thinking straight.' During this visit, he had an argument with his father. He told the family that he thought he should go to the hospital but his father told him not to, saying it was for 'fools'. Mr Daniels then picked up a kitchen knife and stood with it behind the kitchen door. They disarmed him and his father banned him from the parental home, refusing to accept his wife's explanation that their son was ill. Two days before admission his parents came home to find their front door broken down, the furniture smashed or disarranged and their son emptying the kitchen cupboards.

Mrs Daniels could give no other information, saying that she only saw her son occasionally, when he visited. She had not, however, thought his mood was more depressed than normal, nor had she noted any weight loss. She reported that he had a previous hospital admission, and the notes were sent for.

The discharge letter to the GP stated that the previous admission had followed a three-month illness characterized by religiosity, aggressiveness (he had tried to strangle his sister), the belief that he was a person with special powers and the perception of a smell of rotten pork emanating from other people. He had pyrexia on this admission too, but no physical abnormality had been found after intensive investigations. The illness cleared up quite quickly with chlorpromazine, leaving few side effects and, because of a history of cannabis use, a diagnosis of 'possible drug-induced psychosis' was made.

It was decided to admit Mr Daniels to the intensive care ward for observation.

## Preliminary assessment

The first priority in the successful treatment of a patient is to establish the right kind of relationship. The doctor's courtesy, fellow feeling and confidence in the value of psychiatric treatment can help allay apprehension

DEVELOPING A NARRATIVE – MR DANIELS / 39

even in a patient as apparently uncooperative as Mr Daniels. Only after this has been done is the next step possible, which is to obtain all the information necessary for accurate diagnosis and successful treatment. Getting this information may take time. For example, the staff only discovered a month after Mr Daniel's admission that his comment that half his brain was linked to the moon was part of a more complex belief that a war was being fought out inside his head between God in the right side of his brain, and the Devil in the other.

Usually a good deal of information about the patient is necessary for optimal psychiatric treatment. This is because disorder may be manifest in many areas of functioning which all need to be checked, because personal factors, such as constitution, character and social relationships, influence the expression of disorder, and because these factors also influence the choice of treatment and the prognosis.

This reliance on historical information in psychiatry means that careful record-keeping is particularly important. We have found the following principles useful:

- Clearly indicate whether reports are of observations, for example the fact that Mr Daniels had sworn, or judgments, for example that this was 'a sure sign of illness'.

- Either present information clearly as a report that needs checking, or make a definite judgment that the information is accurate. Accuracy may be checked by comparison with another account or estimated by using such characteristics as consistency, credibility and objectivity. Information known to be false may still sometimes be of value as, for example, when it demonstrates delusional memory or the character of a social relationship.

- Separate information about history and mental state. The history documents how the present state has been reached, but the mental state examination provides selected information about the present situation. Observations made by the psychiatrist should therefore be put into the latter category. This category will also contain reports about the person's experiences, but only if they describe the present or immediate past condition, if they are thought to be accurate and if they are relevant to certain areas of psychological function.

- Provide a separate account of the physical state.

- Put historical information into categories, each incorporating like information, such as 'Complaints' or 'History of the Present Illness'. We will follow the format used in standard psychiatric textbooks.

- Order information within categories chronologically.

- Summarize information, whenever this can be done, without making unwarranted assumptions.

- Record the history obtained from other informants separately, quoting the informant's name, relationship to the patient and means of contacting him or her. The information from several sources can be combined later, in the assessment.

The emphasis of the history will vary according to the individual situation. A careful history of previous occupation and social relationships will be necessary in someone who is suspected of having a personality disorder, but may be much less important in an elderly person with dementia; on the other hand detailed information about the physical layout of their accommodation may be essential in the latter case, but not in the former. The importance of the personal context of psychiatric disorder has already been mentioned and is a consistent theme throughout this book. Individual psychiatrists also place a slightly different emphasis on what information to collect. For example, some will stress early life experiences, others family interaction, whilst others again will want information about more remote family members who may have had psychiatric disorders. However, experience has shown that experienced psychiatrists of every persuasion enquire into broad areas of relevance to diagnosis or treatment. Adopting a particular organizational scheme by learning the sequence of sub-headings, such as 'complaints' or 'sexual history', of which it is composed and then using them consistently, is a useful way to ensure that enquiry is systematically carried out in each of these areas.

Most interviews begin with informants giving an account of the problem in the sequence that seems most natural to them. Once they have unburdened themselves it is usually necessary to ask specific questions, and these can follow the same order of topics that will be used in writing down the information. This enables the interviewer to be more attentive rather than worry about which questions to put next. Also, since the order of questions is constructed to make sense of the person's present situation, the sequence in which they are put often offers a welcome reassurance to patients that the psychiatrist is trying to get a complete understanding of their problems.

It is almost always useful to collect information from another source and from further questioning to supplement the initial history. This will be especially important where this is crucial to the diagnosis or the management. These are some of the main sources:

- Previous notes; medical records from other hospitals or the general practitioner; and reports, such as from school.

- Other informants who can give useful information. This will often be a close relative, but may include a flatmate, a neighbour or an employer.

- Observation of, and generally 'getting to know', the person over a period of time.

- Further factual information obtained from the individual.

It is important to collate this information so that important details do not get overlooked. Here again a standard organizational schema, as used in the history, is useful. Collation may also uncover discrepancies. Usually these arise because of some misunderstanding on the part of the psychiatrist, but sometimes they can be due to deliberate or inadvertent misinformation.

One purpose of organizing these reports is to reveal those areas of doubt that can be clarified in subsequent interviews. The complete psychiatric history cannot be attended to at the same time. If it is organized, however, the information will be ordered into categories that build on one another, with facts within each category generally being organized chronologically. The history is then like a narrative. The reader, or listener, can attend to the 'line' or 'paragraph' that is current and even though earlier paragraphs become hazy they will have provided enough preparation and background for the current paragraph to be understood and assimilated.

When the history is 'pre-digested' in this fashion it enables someone who is hearing or reading it for the first time to grasp the essential ingredients of the story, as it unravels. The narrative quality of a well-organized history improves the quality of communication because it provides a sense of a person's development, the impact of vicissitudes and, occasionally, some incoherence in the narrative points to a hitherto undisclosed event or influence.

It is also the logic of the narrative that determines the order of the sub-headings of the history. Any particular moment of a patient's history develops out of earlier events and experiences with which the psychiatrist first needs to become acquainted. The family history therefore precedes the personal history, because knowing about previous generations is helpful in understanding the present one. The complaints and sometimes the history of the present illness come first because, like the introduction to a book, these state the purpose of the enquiry. The description of personality comes at the end of the history, just before the mental state, because this is, in a sense, a summary of certain regularities in the previous history, and is another lens through which the current mental state is viewed.

The process of organizing a history is particularly well illustrated by Mr Daniels, who was unable to give a history in the first week of his admission. Information was therefore obtained in a piecemeal and uncoordinated fashion. We anticipate that our readers will either find this history difficult to grasp as presented, or will begin to organize it for themselves so as to get at the essential facts.

## Further information

Mr Daniels had first been in hospital one year before, when he complained that people smelled like rotten pork and believed that he had special powers. He had no previous serious physical illnesses. He had similar thoughts on his present admission, occasionally thinking that people smelled like dead pigs and that he was one of the few chosen to have a special mark on his forehead (actually a self-inflicted abrasion). He also believed that his breathing had altered and that his body had changed from 'soft' to 'strong'. He thought that people around him were 'the Devil' and that the Devil was trying to gain control of one half of his brain, which was linked to the moon.

Mr Daniels' mother was a 48-year-old laundry worker who had several admissions to a psychiatric hospital with a diagnosis of schizophrenia. She continued to have fluphenazine depot injections. She reported that Mr Daniels had a normal full-term birth in Guyana, and had pneumonia in infancy. She returned to work when he was 12 months old and when he was 3 came to England to join her husband, a 52-year-old caretaker. The couple had five other children: Joyce, aged 23, an unmarried mother; Winston, 18; Pat, 16; Stella, 15; and John, 9. The three youngest children were still at home.

His maternal grandmother brought up Mr Daniels until he was nine, when he joined his parents in the UK. He did not attend school in Guyana and could not write when he went to English secondary school. He did well in a remedial class but was unable to find work after leaving school. Eventually he did a carpentry course and got a job as a carpenter, but was sacked after ten days. His only subsequent work had been in a hospital rehabilitation unit.

Before his previous admission he became very interested in Rastafarianism and then Islam. He smoked cannabis heavily, but said he had not done so before the present admission. When he was examined he was sweaty, feverish and had a tachycardia. He was initially mute, but when he began to speak it was apparent that he was fully orientated and there was no evidence of any cognitive abnormality. Routine drug screening was negative. He said he wasn't hearing voices. His sleep was disturbed, but there was no other evidence of mood disturbance. He said that people could look through his forehead into his brain but that they could not read or interfere with his thoughts. However, on another occasion he said that the Devil could switch on his left-hand 'evil' brain at will. When first admitted he did not answer questions, except to shout 'no'. His behaviour was unpredictable. For example, he suddenly ran down the ward and kicked the entrance door. Mr Daniels gave few details about the time leading up to this admission, and his mother gave the history already described. She and Mr Daniels seemed to get on well although she worried that he never had a girlfriend and thought that her husband was too hard on him. She was worried about his violent and unpredictable behaviour.

This information is included in a systematic fashion in the reassessment presented here.

## Reassessment

Mr Daniels was referred by staff of the day centre because of disturbed behaviour.

## Presenting complaint

(This information was obtained from his mother and the day centre staff, because Mr Daniels was mute on presentation.)

He appeared well until two weeks before admission, when he had seemed restless. One week before, there were 'definite signs of relapse' and he threatened his father. He said he wanted to come back to the hospital at this time. At the day centre he began to say that half his brain was linked to the moon. Two days before admission he smashed furniture at his parents' home, and just before admission he disrupted a staff meeting at the day centre.

## Family history

Mr Daniels' mother is a 48-year-old laundry worker. She came to the UK with his father when he was aged 3. She is currently under treatment for schizophrenia. His father is a 52-year-old caretaker. He has a conflictual relationship with his son. Mr Daniels' siblings are: Joyce, 23, who is unmarried with a baby daughter, and shares a flat with him; Winston, 18, and unmarried; Pat, 16; Stella, 15; John, 9. The three youngest live at home with their parents.

There is no other family member with a psychiatric disorder.

## Personal history

Mr Daniels was born in 1966 in Guyana, following a full-term, normal delivery. He was brought up by his maternal grandmother from 12 months old until aged 9, when he came to live with his parents in an inner city area in a large northern city.

*Education.* Age 11–16: comprehensive school. Remedial class. Age 17: three-month course in carpentry.

*Occupation.* Age 17: ten days as a carpenter. Sacked because of rudeness. None since.

*Sexual history.* No heterosexual relationship. Nothing else known.

*Drug use.* Heavy use of cannabis aged 16, but not recently.

## Past medical history

Pneumonia, aged nine months. Pyrexia of unknown origin, aged 16.

## Past psychiatric history

He had a psychotic illness aged 16, following a three-month history of religious preoccupations and heavy cannabis use. Olfactory hallucinations and grandiose ideas were noted at this time.

## Previous personality

No information was available.

## Mental state examination

*Appearance and general behaviour*

On admission he was dishevelled and looked suspicious and did not cooperate with the examination. During his first admission his behaviour was described as 'explosive' with sudden outbursts of violent activity.

## Speech

He was initially mute, and then shouted 'no' when asked to do anything. Later, he began to talk spontaneously and eventually answered questions promptly and sensibly.

## Mood

He was neither depressed nor elated. There was no disturbance of appetite. His total sleep time was reduced.

## Thought content

He was preoccupied with his abnormal ideas.

## Abnormal beliefs and interpretations of events

He believed that he was one of the chosen few, that an abrasion on his forehead demonstrated this and that his bodily functions have altered. He thought that his brain could be 'looked into' but did not think his thoughts could be read. He also believed that one or other side of his brain could be switched on or off by the Devil.

## Abnormal experiences

He had occasional olfactory hallucinations (the smell of a dead pig coming from people). He said he did not have any auditory hallucinations.

## Cognitive state

His orientation was normal. No abnormality was detected in his attention, concentration and memory. His intelligence was low or low to average.

## Self-appraisal

He was convinced of the reality of his experiences.

## Physical examination

He was reluctant to be examined. He was sweating and there was an abrasion on his forehead. His temperature was 38.5°C, and his pulse was 120 per minute, full and regular.

We have now reached the stage where subsequent chapters of this book will begin. In doing so, we have shown how disparate information can be organized into a clinical narrative. This is the first step towards producing an overall assessment, or formulation, of the psychiatric problem in the context of individuals, their lives and their experiences.

These assessments are a further step in our organization of information. They contain what psychiatrists keep in mind from the full summary because it seems most important to their management. The ability to make the right selection, or inference, is one of the essential skills of psychiatry and is dependent on context and individual circumstances. However, we have found that reassessments are required in order to answer three closely related questions:

- Are there any misleading gaps in the information?

- Is there any information that is doubtful?

- What are the psychiatric implications of this information?

The psychiatrist now needs to consider whether more information is required, whether the information available needs further clarification and what is the possible diagnosis, treatment and prognosis.

It has been said that most psychiatrists make a diagnosis within two minutes of starting an interview. Sometimes they do so even earlier while, for example, reading the referral letter. This is probably inevitable. We have found it helpful to see a diagnosis made in this way as a tentative hypothesis, which needs to be tested during the interview. This not only makes taking a history a much more active and enquiring process, it is also reassuring if something unexpected or urgent happens, because the interviewer has ready a view of the underlying problem. We have tried to show in subsequent chapters how an initial assessment changes as further information becomes available.

We end this chapter with a provisional assessment of Mr Daniels' illness. Although sketchy, it was valuable when Mr Daniels absconded shortly after admission, because it enabled the staff to recognize that he was both psychotic and a danger to others and so led to effective action.

## Assessment

### Diagnosis

Mr Daniels is psychotic. Although mute on admission, he was not stuporose and was found not to be confused when this could be conclusively tested. An acute brain syndrome, which may have been suggested by his pyrexia, can therefore be ruled out. There are no features of an affective disorder, but there are many features of schizophrenia, including a delusion of passivity. Schizophrenia, or a schizophreniform illness, is therefore the most likely diagnosis.

### Aetiology

Mr Daniels has both a family history of schizophrenia and a previous history of an illness similar to the present one. It should therefore be assumed that he has a long-standing vulnerability to schizophrenia. The previous illness was associated with heavy cannabis use, and may have been drug-induced. The immediate history is against drug-induction of this illness, but this cannot yet be excluded.

The marked pyrexia suggests an occult physical disorder of which the schizophrenia may be a symptom. However, despite extensive investigations no disorder was found on the previous admission, when Mr Daniels was also pyrexial. It is possible that the pyrexia on this occasion is a manifestation of an unusually severe degree of the inflammatory response that often occurs in the first few days of an acute psychosis.

The conflict in Mr Daniels' family during the early part of his illness suggests that family factors may be important in explaining the severity of his breakdown.

*Further information*

More information on Mr Daniels' recent drug use needs to be obtained. His physical state needs to be thoroughly investigated. Other precipitants of this present illness, such as stresses in his home situation or recent life events, should not be neglected whilst these investigations are progressing since several synergistic factors may have been active. Even though he has left home, his family may still be an important source of support and their attitude to him and to his illness will need to be investigated.

*Management*

Mr Daniels has been violent before admission, and inpatient treatment is indicated. Antipsychotic treatment has been effective in the past and is likely to be so again. Little would be gained by further observation without medication. This would probably increase the risk of violence on the ward and would also add unnecessary difficulty to the task of making a relationship and obtaining a thorough history from him.

If he initially refuses treatment every attempt should be made to persuade him otherwise before a compulsory treatment order, which would be applicable in this case, is invoked. Further treatment should be based on the determination of the cause of the present illness.

*Prognosis*

The prognosis for this episode is likely to be good, as it was for the previous episode. Longer-term prognosis will depend on the eventual diagnosis, the effectiveness of treatment and Mr Daniels' capacity to cooperate.

# Chapter 3

# *Assessing Suicidal Risk*

## *Mr Wrigley*

### Presenting complaint

Mr Wrigley was referred for an urgent outpatient assessment by his general practitioner. The letter said, 'He is suffering from anxiety, depression and has suicidal tendencies. He wanted to assault himself with a knife last April [five months earlier] …his depression is getting worse and I am quite concerned about him.'

Mr Wrigley was seen on his own and complained that he was a 'whole mass of nerves' and that he 'just can't keep still'. He said he was 'stopping away from people' which was 'not like me'. This all started after his retirement on medical grounds. Two years before the interview he had 'a stroke' affecting his right side. He made a good recovery, but then, two months later, he had another on his left side leaving him with a weak arm and leg. Although it 'soon wore off' he had to give up his job as a hospital porter because he was incapable of heavy lifting. No alternative employment was available and he was made redundant.

Mr Wrigley felt he had increasingly 'changed' after that. He began to burst into tears over nothing, he had to force himself to eat because he had no appetite for food and he slept for shorter and shorter periods at night. He lost interest in sex, and had not had sexual intercourse with his wife for 18 months before the interview. His wife had taken to sleeping in a separate bed because of his restlessness at night.

Mr Wrigley described the reported attempt on his life as follows. He had been having tea with his daughter, his wife, and her sister when he picked up a knife from the table and made as if to stab himself with it. He then burst into anguished tears when he was restrained, and sobbed, 'I'm sorry, I'm sorry.'

His general practitioner had treated him with benzodiazepines but Mr Wrigley felt little benefit from them. He had been told he could not drink alcohol whilst taking them. Since he felt that it was not manly to drink soft drinks, he had avoided social occasions and so became more socially isolated.

## Family history

Mr Wrigley had no memories of his father, who died when he was one year old. His mother died some years before the onset of this illness. He described her as a capable, humorous and cheerful lady. He was originally the youngest of three children. His brother died of a brain tumour at the age of 24, when Mr Wrigley was 19, and his sister died of cancer a few months before the interview.

There was no family history of psychiatric disorder or epilepsy.

## Personal history

Mr Wrigley had a happy childhood. He was born and brought up in a close, but impoverished area of inner London. He enjoyed school, and left at 14 without qualifications. He found work immediately after leaving school and was continuously employed in various jobs, excluding a period of national service, until his early retirement. His occupations had all involved labouring or assembly work.

He married when he was 28 and had two children, a son and a daughter. He described his marriage as happy. He lived in a council flat with his wife and daughter.

## Past medical history

He had two recent cerebrovascular episodes as already described, but could not recall any other serious illness, including epilepsy.

## Past psychiatric history

Mr Wrigley had a period of inpatient treatment while he was undergoing his national service. It was assumed that this was associated with depression following the death of his brother.

## Previous personality

Mr Wrigley's account of himself suggested that before his illness he was optimistic, active and sociable with no tendency to get depressed.

## Mental state examination

### Appearance and general behaviour

Mr Wrigley was a tall, notably thin man who showed no spontaneous movements and whose face was set in an expression of both sadness and apprehension. He seemed often on the point of tears.

### Speech

He spoke slowly and with no tonal modulation. He was markedly slow in replying to questions. His answers were to the point but terse.

### Mood

Mr Wrigley appeared and felt agitated and miserable. There was nothing he enjoyed and he had to force himself to eat. He had lost over 14 lbs in weight since the beginning of his illness. He lay awake for up to two hours after going to bed at night and usually woke again after two or three hours and was then unable to get back to sleep. He had lost interest in all his customary activities (betting, sing-song evenings at the club and gardening at home) but his energy was little affected and he spent a great deal of his day on long solitary walks. He reported difficulty in concentrating and could not sit and watch television. He also had difficulty in remembering things;

for example, the names of friends and the words of songs. He had lost all interest in sex.

Mr Wrigley said that he felt that life was not worth living. He had wished to die and occasionally thought of ending his life, but had made no plans to do so and said that he had no current intention of ending his life.

### Thought content

Mr Wrigley had vague worries about his health. His main preoccupation was with his lost work. He felt that he would never have become ill if he had only stayed at work.

### Abnormal beliefs and interpretations of events

None were elicited.

### Abnormal experiences

None were elicited.

### Cognitive state

Mr Wrigley knew where he was being interviewed. He also knew the day, month and year, although not the date. His recall of a name and address after five minutes was perfect. Mr Wrigley was asked about current news items and accurately reported two.

### Self-appraisal

Mr Wrigley said, 'My nerves have been affected by my inability to adapt to retirement.'

## Physical examination

This was not performed at the time.

A brief collateral history was obtained from his wife and youngest daughter, who had accompanied him to his appointment. They confirmed the broad outlines of his history, and of his previous personality. Mrs

Wrigley wanted her husband 'to have some treatment'. She was angry with her general practitioner for his reluctance to refer her husband to a psychiatrist earlier. This referral had only come about, she said, because she had 'threatened to go private'.

Neither Mr nor Mrs Wrigley wanted him to come into hospital.

## Preliminary assessment

Mr Wrigley is a 59-year-old retired hospital porter who was seen in the outpatient department at the urgent request of his general practitioner. He is a married man with two children, the younger of whom still lives with his wife and himself. He was born and brought up in the local area. His father died when he was aged one. His brother died when he was 20 and, recently, his sister. He was briefly 'depressed' after his brother died but had no other psychiatric illness and appears to have been a consistently cheerful and sociable man.

Two years previously he had a stroke involving his right side, and subsequently another stroke affecting his left side, which resulted in his being retired from work on medical grounds. Since then he has become increasingly preoccupied with his loss and has come to regard the future with hopelessness. Over the last 18 months he has lost a considerable amount of weight and he has also suffered from increasingly disturbed sleep, marked by waking early in the morning. His personality has changed considerably, in that he has gradually given up his interests and has avoided meeting other people. He made a suicide attempt five months previously.

On examination, he was anxious and dejected. He was retarded in speech but his concentration and memory were not clinically impaired and he was not deluded or hallucinated. He has thought of ending his life but has no plans to do so.

### Diagnosis

It is clear that Mr Wrigley is depressed. He manifests psychological, somatic (biological) and cognitive features of depression. The range and intensity of these features fulfil both the ICD10 and DSMIV criteria for a 'severe depressive episode without psychotic features'. His previous hospitalization raises the possibility that this could be classified as a *recurrent* depressive illness. Uppermost in the psychiatrist's mind, in assessing a depressed, unemployed man in late middle age, will be the risk of suicide. This issue should be addressed in the initial management plan, particularly since there was a history of deliberate self-harm.

Some degree of depression is understandable, although by no means inevitable, after severe illness. However, this should not prevent the diagnosis of a depressive disorder. It is unlikely that Mr Wrigley's depressive symptoms can be attributed only to a *prolonged depressive reaction*, whether to his stroke, or his redundancy, or both. DSMIV criteria require the onset of emotional symptoms to be within three months of the stressor (within one month for the ICD10). This might be met by the second stroke or by his redundancy. However, *adjustment reactions* do not continue beyond six months according to DSMIV (up to two years in the case of mild depression, according to ICD10) and should not fulfil criteria for a major depressive episode. Furthermore, the symptoms do not increase in severity, as have Mr Wrigley's. His state has not improved with the passage of time, or following recovery from his strokes. This is all evidence in favour of Mr Wrigley having a depressive illness rather than a depressive adjustment reaction.

## Aetiology

Three types of aetiological factors need to be considered: predisposing, provoking and exacerbating factors. It is convenient to divide these into constitutional and psychosocial components.

Since relatively little personal information is available about Mr Wrigley none of the possible aetiological factors can be ruled out at this stage and each of them will therefore be considered.

### CONSTITUTIONAL PREDISPOSITION

Most people will become depressed if subjected to sufficient stress. However, a few have a hereditary disposition to do so more severely, or in response to less extreme challenges. Mr Wrigley gives little evidence of such vulnerability. He provided no family history of depression or 'depressive spectrum' disorder such as alcoholism, which occurs more commonly in relatives of patients with a hereditary predisposition to depression. Neither does he have a depressive, anankastic or cyclothymic personality, which may also be associated.

PSYCHOSOCIAL PREDISPOSITION

The details of Mr Wrigley's early upbringing so far available are insufficiently detailed to assess its contribution. It has been suggested that individuals who have lost a parent by death in infancy, as has Mr Wrigley, are more likely to develop depression in later life.

CONSTITUTIONAL PROVOCATION

Mr Wrigley is known to have suffered a stroke, which is known to provoke depression. Having a stroke is frightening in the short term and may cause grief in the longer term, because of the loss of physical function that it causes. However, depression may also be a direct consequence of neurological impairment, particularly when this involves limbic structures.

PSYCHOSOCIAL PROVOCATION

Although a wide variety of life-experiences, or 'life events', may provoke depression, those involving threat or loss appear to be the most noxious. Mr Wrigley has experienced 3 major events involving loss – his redundancy, his stroke and the later loss of his sister – and the stroke also carries with it a threat of future serious disability or death. Each of these events could have many subsidiary consequences, and these, too, may provoke further depression. One example given by Mr Wrigley is that he engaged less on one of his principal sources of pleasure, going to 'the club' with his friends, because he was ashamed of being redundant and because he had difficulty in remembering the words of the songs that were sung in the bar.

CONSTITUTIONAL EXACERBATION

This may have an indirect effect and in Mr Wrigley's case it relates to his stroke. Any persistent disability may restrict or prevent activities that would normally be recuperative. Very little is known about his physical state but it is known that his stroke lost him his job and that unemployment generally results in a reduced ability to cope with adversity.

PSYCHOSOCIAL EXACERBATION

This includes an individual's coping strategies and resources. It is not known which strategies Mr Wrigley used to surmount difficulty, nor what help was available to him through relationships with other people, notably his wife. However, if much of Mr Wrigley's self-esteem and the esteem of others derive from his skills at doing a job and earning a wage, then he is likely to have coped worse with both redundancy and physical disability than someone who experiences him- or herself as valued for some other attribute, such as sensitivity to others.

## Management
GENERAL ISSUES

More information is needed to determine the aetiology of Mr Wrigley's illness. In a first outpatient interview it is difficult to obtain a comprehensive history. More details about his family and his life will be necessary in order to test some of the aetiological hypotheses already mentioned. The diagnosis of manic-depressive psychosis could be more confidently ruled out if this failed to reveal evidence of a manic-depressive diathesis. It will be necessary for example to enquire further about the emotional atmosphere in Mr Wrigley's family of origin, their material circumstances, and his memories of, or thoughts about, his father, and about his reaction to his mother's death. It might also be helpful to know how often he saw his sister, so that the closeness of the family can be assessed.

Further enquiry needs to be made about his neurological disability since the strokes. He therefore needs more detailed cognitive testing and a physical examination. A brain scan may be indicated to determine the location and extent of the cerebral lesions.

Mr Wrigley's ability to cope needs to be assessed. It is convenient to do this by considering his personal, social and material resources separately. His personal history is likely to be a particularly good gauge of the former. How he responded to previous losses and how he tried to combat the depression in its early stages are two considerations. His major social resources are his wife and his friends at the club. Some assessment needs to be made of the present quality of these relationships, and how much support Mr Wrigley feels he receives from them. Something needs to be known about his home, such as whether he owns it and how satisfactory it is to him, and his contact with his neighbours. It would also be useful to enquire specifically about his financial situation, including possible debts.

The timing of the events leading up to Mr Wrigley's illness needs to be checked against the development of his symptoms, since this will give crucial information about which of the possible factors precipitated his depressive illness.

The additional information so far considered is not essential to immediate management, and can therefore be obtained at a later date. However, some information relevant to this is missing, and is considered in the next section.

IMMEDIATE MANAGEMENT

The most pressing problem is whether or not Mr Wrigley should come into hospital in order to expedite his treatment, to relieve his distress and, most urgently, to prevent suicide or serious self-harm resulting from a failed suicide attempt. The answer depends on the characteristics of Mr Wrigley's illness, his intentions, his previous behaviour, and his personal situation.

The first step in the management is therefore to review these characteristics, especially those that are risk factors for suicide, and to enquire further about those whose presence is still undetermined.

INTENTIONS AND PREVIOUS BEHAVIOUR

Mr Wrigley was clear that he had considered suicide but had made no plans to do so. Considerable importance is usually attached to a patient's intentions, and supplementary questions such as 'Have you ever thought how you would kill yourself?' should also be put. There are indications that Mr Wrigley minimizes his symptoms, possibly because he feels that he 'shouldn't have' suicidal ideas. Even if Mr Wrigley stated his intentions correctly, the weight to put on them will depend on his personality. Conscientious people may deliberate for some time about suicide, but impulsive ones may kill themselves with as little forethought as they have lived.

The fact that Mr Wrigley has made a previous suicide attempt during the course of the illness is, by contrast, a definite risk factor that should therefore be set against his stated intention not to do so again. Not enough of the circumstances of this attempt are known to be able to assess its seriousness. The exact details need to be enquired into, and it would also be useful to ask the relatives about any other attempts at, or apparent preparations for, suicide.

PERSONAL SITUATION

There are a number of important risk factors that apply to Mr Wrigley; in particular his age and sex, because suicide and the presence of a physical illness are most common in men over 50. His lack of employment also increases the risk, especially since work has, in the past, been a source of both pride and satisfaction to him.

Mr Wrigley's close ties with family and friends are protective factors. However, he has apparently withdrawn socially following the development of his depression. It is therefore important to establish how much contact he presently has with others, how satisfying this is to him, and how protective these relationships are. It is particularly important to assess the present quality of his relationship with his wife. This should be done tactfully, but in some depth; for example, by asking about what they do together, whether they have common interests, when they last had a row, what it was about, and when they last had any physical contact. There are therefore many factors in Mr Wrigley's situation whose cumulative effect may well make the risk of suicide a significant one.

The fact that Mr Wrigley is unwell, that there is an effective treatment, that he is likely to get better more quickly in hospital than at home, and that there are risks to his safety if he remains at home, are all indications for admission to hospital. The risk of suicide is also likely to be reduced by hospital admission: first, because Mr Wrigley could be supervised more closely by nursing staff; second, because he might find it easier to disclose suicidal ideas to emotionally neutral, professional care-givers who are experienced at recognizing the indications of a suicide attempt, which may sometimes be subtle; and third, more active treatment can be instituted. Hospital admission would also have the advantage that Mr Wrigley would be removed from any psychosocial factors that aggravate his depression, such as the criticism from families which commonly occurs in response to long-standing irritability or social withdrawal.

Mr and Mrs Wrigley are both unhappy about the possibility of admission. Mrs Wrigley may feel that she has failed her husband, and Mr Wrigley that he is inadequate or incurable. These, and other worries, must be discussed. They are also likely to want to know about the alternatives to inpatient treatment, such as day hospital or outpatient attendance or, if available, 24-hour crisis management.

ADMISSION

Mr Wrigley has suffered from a long illness. His suicide attempt occurred five months before his outpatient appointment, and has not been repeated. Should neither he nor his wife be willing for him to come into hospital, the immediate risk to him is not sufficient to justify compulsory admission. However, he is ill enough, and the longer-term risk is great enough, for regular, frequent reassessment to be indicated. A community psychiatric nurse could provide this effectively by monitoring his mental state at home and liaising with the community psychiatrist, who can review his progress on a regular basis. He might also be a good candidate for day hospital treatment, where this is available.

Regular reassessment would impress Mr Wrigley with the psychiatrist's concern; it would enable him to build up a consistent relationship with the psychiatric nurse and the psychiatrist, and to acclimatize himself to the hospital. It would also help the psychiatrist to gain a more thorough understanding of Mr Wrigley and his illness.

The psychiatrist should advise Mr and Mrs Wrigley to contact him, or a named member of the community mental health team, immediately should there be any deterioration in Mr Wrigley's condition, and should also give them an alternative person to contact, if unavailable.

Compulsory admission will need to be reconsidered if Mr Wrigley's symptoms worsen or if he expresses suicidal ideas, and he continues to refuse hospital admission. It should also be considered if Mr Wrigley fails to maintain contact.

TREATMENT

Once the circumstances in which Mr Wrigley is to be treated have been established the specific elements of the treatment can be considered. The first of these is physical treatment.

At this stage, antidepressant medication is the treatment of first choice, and is likely to be effective. The dose can be built up more rapidly and side effects monitored more easily if Mr Wrigley is an inpatient, or if he attends the hospital frequently. A sedative antidepressant of proven efficacy but safe in overdose would be best, with the dose being given at night to help him sleep. He could also be offered a less sedative antidepressant with a non-benzodiazepine hypnotic for extra night sedation. Mr and Mrs Wrigley should be told that antidepressants may cause a transient worsening of mood shortly after they are begun, and that they take at least two weeks to be fully effective. Patients who respond to antidepressants may become more energetic before they become less depressed. The risk of suicide may consequently be greater during this period, and even more careful supervision necessary.

The risk of suicide must be discussed with Mrs Wrigley and possible warning signs, such as the expression of suicidal ideas, a worsening of his mood or, paradoxically, a sudden elation, should be mentioned.

The alternative physical option is electro-convulsive therapy (ECT), which is at least as effective in psychotic depression as drug treatment, and usually quicker. It is contra-indicated, however, if Mr Wrigley's strokes were due to hypertension or bleeding from a vascular malformation and should not therefore be given until Mr Wrigley has been more thoroughly investigated physically. It is also unwise to give the first-ever ECT on an outpatient basis.

Psychological treatments such as cognitive-behavioural treatment (CBT) have been demonstrated to be as effective as antidepressant treatments in mild to moderate depressive illness. However, the clinical psychologist in the community team had at least one month's waiting list for assessments, which was too long for Mr Wrigley's current situation. This should not preclude the community nurse or psychiatrist helping Mrs Wrigley to talk over her feelings about the situation, which might alleviate potential sources of tension between them. Follow-up visits could also be used to identify and challenge some of his gloomy depressive ruminations – for example, that he has been on the 'scrap heap' since he lost his job.

## Further details

Mr Wrigley could not be persuaded to come into hospital and made light of his depression. He was allocated a community nurse who saw him twice-weekly and an outpatient appointment arranged for two weeks later. A serotonin specific reuptake inhibitor (SSRI), paroxetine, was started, with a hypnotic, zopiclone, at night.

The community nurse found little change in this mental state over the two weeks. On the day that he was due to be seen by his psychiatrist Mr Wrigley cut his throat and both his wrists with a blade from a safety razor. He left the following note on two blank pages torn out of a book.

> To Dorris [wife] and Tracey [daughter]
>
> I just can't take any more of this misery I feel and I am making your life and Tracey's a misery too. That is the way I feel from morning till night. I've had enough so I'm getting out of it. I am sorry love. That is the way I feel. I leave the money in the bank to you Dorris. And the money upstairs under my shirts. I can't take any more Dorris. Nor can you. If we can't live happy it's NO GOOD. I'm making life A MISERY for you and Tracey. I'm sorry, good bye love. I want to be cremated Dorris.
>
> PS Tell Lofty and my other mates that they're THE BEST FRIENDS anyone could have.

He was semi-conscious when his daughter discovered him. In hospital he was found to have severed his long flexor tendons and his ulnar artery in his left wrist, and to have incised his larynx. Other vital structures had been missed, as often occurs if the throat is cut when the neck is extended. The skin of his right wrist was cut in a number of places but deeper structures were untouched. Mr Wrigley's systolic blood pressure on admission was sixty. He was resuscitated and an emergency tracheotomy was performed. The severed tendons were repaired and his wounds sutured. An in-dwelling urinary catheter was also inserted.

Mr Wrigley's physical condition improved rapidly and four days after admission he was seen by the same psychiatrist who had seen him at the initial assessment. He began by apologizing for what he had done, and said, 'It wasn't your fault.' He was sorry that he had failed and wanted to be dead, but 'would never do that again. Not after all the work you doctors have done'. He was transferred to the psychiatric unit shortly after, and the nurse accompanying him reported that he was 'much better' and was smiling. Mr Wrigley's convalescence was uneventful, apart from an acute exacerbation of his chronic bronchitis, which responded to physiotherapy and antibiotics. His most persistent physical complaint was the weakness of his right hand.

The nursing staff were particularly anxious about Mr Wrigley making another suicide attempt. When asked whether he had any intention to do so he would say 'I think I've done enough damage' and then smile or make a joke. He was seen to bang his right hand on furniture and described his physical condition as 'rubbish'. On one visit by his wife and daughter he alarmed them by picking up a knife and stroking its edge with his thumb for several minutes.

Mr Wrigley's antidepressant and zopiclone were re-started after his transfer from the surgical ward. Mrs Wrigley and her daughter were interviewed again, and a more detailed history obtained from Mr Wrigley. This took place over three interviews, after his tracheotomy tube had been removed and he could talk without undue strain.

## Additional history

Little new information was obtained about Mr Wrigley's father. He had no memory of him and had never enquired about him. He thought he died in his late 30s and that he had a bad chest and possible TB. His mother died aged 91 from 'old age'. His younger sister, who had died earlier that year, had a 'nervous breakdown' in the 1950s, but no further information about this was available. She had married when she was 35, had a daughter who emigrated to Australia, and became a widow about ten years previously. He confirmed that his family had always been close. He regularly saw his own children, his sister (until her death) and her daughter, and kept in touch with his sister's son who was in Australia.

Mr Wrigley's various jobs included furnace labouring, and motor mower assembly. After leaving the Water Board, where he was a labourer, he became a hospital porter for ten years. He married at 29 after a courtship of only three months. His wife was four years older than himself. Mrs Wrigley described the marriage as 'generally happy' and said that they had the 'occasional row'. She said that Mr Wrigley had always been affectionate with the children but did not particularly enjoy their company. She described herself as 'nervy' and said that she had recently developed asthma.

Mrs Wrigley usually described her husband as 'daft' when talking about his suicide attempt. She spoke much more than he did in interviews, and on one occasion said, 'I know about depression. No one has been more depressed than I have.'

The Wrigleys' son was 28, and happily married. Tracey, their daughter, was 20, lived at home and had been unemployed since leaving school. Both children were very concerned about their father and visited regularly.

Mr Wrigley was a heavy smoker. He drank most nights and went to the pub several days a week. This had become his main interest in the last few years. His family concurred in saying that before his illness he had been a very sociable, well-liked and equable individual who preferred the company of other men.

Mr Wrigley had been well until his first stroke. Although he then retired, his mood remained cheerful until his second stroke, six months later, when he was investigated by a neurologist. He was found to have increased tone in all four limbs, greater on the left than the right. Aortography showed a common origin of the subclavian carotid arteries but his cardiovascular system was otherwise normal, and he was not hypertensive. An MRI scan showed a small, high intensity area, adjacent to the lateral border of the body of the right ventricle. His general practitioner thought he was 'understandably upset' about losing his job and had been reluctant to treat him. Mr Wrigley reinforced this view by dismissing his psychological symptoms in consultations, which were usually for physical symptoms such as a 'stabbing pain' in his side or 'funny feelings' in his stomach.

A diagnosis of brain-stem ischaemia had been made and Mr Wrigley was discharged on aspirin. He discontinued this believing that he could not drink while taking it. His depressed mood was noted at outpatient follow-up, but his complaints of pain and weight loss were thought to be physical in origin.

### Further progress

Ten days after transfer to the psychiatric unit Mr Wrigley's physical condition was as follows. He was fully mobile. A small sinus remained over the site of his tracheotomy but there was no communication with his trachea. His neck and wrists had healed, and his chest was clear. His cardiovascular system was normal, and he was passing urine without a catheter. Neurological examination revealed no abnormalities of his facial nerves. However, he showed signs of a left upper motor neurone lesion, with significantly reduced power, associated with increased tone and reflexes, in his right, dominant hand. He also had agraphaesthesia and astereognosis of both hands, which was worse on the right than the left. He complained of his right hand being 'dead', but light touch sensation was only mildly impaired, and pinprick sensation was normal.

When he was interviewed at a ward round ten days after transfer, Mr Wrigley looked pale and listless, but his face betrayed little emotion except for a fixedly corrugated forehead and occasional moistening of his eyes. He smiled once or twice in response to his own 'jokes' – for example, when his wife's concern for him was being discussed, he said, 'She's only interested while she doesn't know where I keep my money.'

Mr Wrigley's spirits appeared to improve shortly after his transfer but then sank again, although he still said that he 'was slightly better than last year'. His appetite remained poor, but his sleep had returned to normal. He said 'Not yet' when asked whether he had again thought of ending his life, and he prefaced discussions about living with his family with the proviso, 'If I'm still here.' His mood was consistent throughout the day.

On several occasions Mr Wrigley expressed abnormally suspicious ideas. For example, in a casual conversation in the hospital grounds he said that everyone in his neighbourhood would know of his suicide attempt and, pointing to a postman who happened to be passing, he said, 'He'll tell them all about it.' Mr Wrigley appeared not to dwell on these ideas once they occurred to him, and may even have forgotten them shortly afterwards.

Mr Wrigley continued to experience difficulty with his concentration and his memory; for example, he made many mistakes when attempting to serially subtract 7 from 100.

Mr Wrigley believed that he was depressed and thought that he would never improve.

Following an occupational therapy assessment Mr Wrigley started a limited rehabilitation programme. He wrote off many of the activities as 'no good for a man', but he was drawn to the greenhouse and spoke of his previous skill in the garden. He spoke bitterly of his present 'uselessness', particularly his unemployability, but at the same time berated his employers for not finding him alternative 'light work', because, 'If they had, none of this would have happened.'

His chest X-ray, full blood count, urea, electrolytes, thyroid function tests and ECG were all normal. Syphilis serology was negative.

He continued to take paroxetine, 20mg a day, which had been started when he was an outpatient. His zopiclone was discontinued after his sleep improved, and olanzapine (a major tranquillizer), 10mg at night, was added when he revealed his suspicious beliefs.

## Reassessment

The most important decision at this stage is whether the present treatment has failed to work and, if so, what are the alternatives. The urgency of this decision will depend on how dangerous to himself Mr Wrigley is considered to be, and this requires an accurate reassessment of the severity of his depression.

### Diagnosis

All the evidence, including his nearly fatal suicide attempt, confirms that Mr Wrigley is severely depressed. His occasionally abnormal suspicious ideas are consistent with a *severe depressive episode with psychotic symptoms*

(ICD10), and are *mood congruent* (DSMIV). No previous episode of mania or evidence of cyclothymic or obsessional personality has emerged. Although there is now a family history of 'nervous illness' it is not characteristically depressive. There is therefore no evidence of a bipolar diathesis and this favours the diagnosis of depressive illness.

Mr Wrigley has also developed a spastic paresis associated with sensory loss of his right hand. This cannot have been present before his suicide attempt because he was then able to hold a thin safety razor blade with sufficient strength to sever the tendons of his left wrist.

Two diagnoses therefore need to be considered in formulating Mr Wrigley's management and prognosis: a severe depressive illness with psychotic symptoms, and his recent spastic paresis.

## Aetiology

*Depressive illness with psychotic features.* There is now evidence that Mr Wrigley has a constitutional vulnerability to depression. His family's closeness over the years and his consistently warm accounts of his mother make it unlikely that Mr Wrigley's upbringing left him with a vulnerability to depression. However, it must be stressed that very little is known, even now, of Mr Wrigley's memories, feelings or preconceptions which might give a clue about how his early life shaped his present personality and coping abilities. Any theory of a life-long predisposition to depression would anyway have to explain the late onset of his illness.

It is notable that Mr Wrigley appears not to have become depressed following his first stroke and his consequent redundancy, but only two weeks after his second stroke, which was much less physically disabling. Although it is possible that the six months was an 'incubation period' during which a depressive reaction was building up as Mr Wrigley's emotional resources became exhausted, it seems more probable that the most important precipitant of Mr Wrigley's depression was the second stroke. This is likely to have had psychological significance, as a further reminder of Mr Wrigley's vulnerability. It is also possible that it had a direct neurobiological effect.

Mr Wrigley's unemployment, and an ever-deepening spiral of angry and self-critical ruminations linked to it, could have maintained and aggravated his depression. Although there is a strong undercurrent of anger in his present relationship with his wife, there is no reason to suppose that this was long-standing. Her anger seems an understandable reaction to Mr Wrigley's long, demanding illness and, even more, to the unpleasantness of his suicide attempt. His anger remains unexplained but is equally directed at medical and nursing staff, as evinced by his 'gallows humour'.

Mr Wrigley's depressive illness appears to have been well established by the time his sister died. It is not known whether he had anticipated her death, or whether it also contributed to his depression.

The reason that Mr Wrigley made his suicide attempt when he did remains uncertain, and this increases concern about a future attempt. One possible factor is that he might have become more energetic in response to antidepressant treatment, but a similar response did not occur when the same antidepressant was continued after admission.

*Spastic paresis.* The most likely explanation for this is that an extension of his previous infarct occurred during his episode of haemorrhagic shock.

## Management

There is some information that is important to obtain from every patient. A history of alcohol use is an example. A lot of this information is missing in Mr Wrigley's case. More needs to be known about his drinking habits; and also about his national service, work, sexual, and any forensic history; and about his financial and domestic circumstances. There are also one or two features of Mr Wrigley's history, as of any psychiatric history, that stimulate curiosity. Why, for example, is there such a big age gap between the children? One does not yet know him as a person. This makes the assessment of his disorder, and of further risk of suicide, very difficult.

It has been difficult to gather a fuller history because of his weak physical condition on admission, his depression, and his defensive attitudes towards psychiatry and psychiatrists. Enough of a picture has emerged, however, for several key items of missing information to be considered.

### DEPRESSIVE ILLNESS WITH PSYCHOTIC FEATURES

It appears that Mrs Wrigley has also suffered a psychological illness. The details of this, and its relationship to Mr Wrigley's illness, need clarification. Provided she gives consent, her medical notes should be obtained.

The details of Mr Wrigley's redundancy remain unclear. Was he offered alternative employment, redundancy pay or a pension? Who made the decision?

### SPASTIC PARESIS

Although Mr Wrigley may have suffered a further infarction, it is unlikely that his cerebral cortex has been affected. Nevertheless, his cognitive function should be tested after he has recovered from his depressive illness. A further MRI scan is probably not indicated.

Why did Mr Wrigley try so hard to conceal his illness? Do his friends and family really only value him when he is the 'life and soul' of the party? Does he believe that depression is due to 'weakness'? Is he frightened of psychiatric hospitals? Is he ashamed of being a psychiatric patient? Does he think it unmanly to show feelings?

### SUICIDE RISK

The exact circumstances and antecedents of both of Mr Wrigley's suicide attempts should be ascertained. A careful drinking history needs to be taken. Intoxication may 'release' suicidal behaviour and alcohol dependence itself increases the risk of suicide. Are there any traits of Mr Wrigley's character that may have predisposed him to suicide? What is his attitude to it? Does he have any strong religious beliefs, which include beliefs about suicide?

## Plan

### DEPRESSION – THE ACUTE EPISODE

Since Mr Wrigley has not been taking his antidepressant continuously, it cannot be certain that he has failed to respond. However, his sense of hopelessness and distress, and staff fears for his safety, are compelling reasons for changing the treatment. Mr Wrigley is receiving a standard dose (20mg) of paroxetine. The alternatives are to increase the dose of antidepressant, switch to another class of antidepressant (such as a tricyclic), add lithium, which has a demonstrated augmentation effect in refractory depression, or to use ECT. In view of the fears for his safety ECT was considered the treatment of choice. It is likely to be at least as effective as an antidepressant and probably acts sooner. It is not contra-indicated by Mr Wrigley's stroke since this was not a complication of hypertension. Mr Wrigley's tracheotomy was a contra-indication, but this has now healed, and his physical condition is satisfactory.

It is also important to try and reduce Mr Wrigley's self-condemnation and sense of worthlessness. His sense of grievance and the hostility associated with his depression have probably contributed to both of these. They can be made more tolerable if they are 'contained' by nursing and medical staff by being listened to, but not argued away. An attempt should also be made to raise Mr Wrigley's self-esteem by providing him with activities that he finds satisfying. In view of his interest in woodwork the occupational therapist should be consulted about incorporating this as part of his daily routine.

Mr Wrigley's family should be encouraged to maintain their visits, given the opportunity to express their anxieties, and reassured that they were not to blame for his illness or for the suicide attempt.

DEPRESSION – THE LONG TERM

Whilst the circumstances that contributed to Mr Wrigley's depression still obtain, there is a risk it will recur. To prevent this an attempt should therefore be made to alter those that are of aetiological importance; for example, by providing Mr Wrigley with some occupation. Re-employment is unlikely, in view of his physical state, age and lack of marketable skills, but voluntary work or a day centre are possibilities. The choice would depend on their availability and acceptability to Mr Wrigley. It would be important to suggest an activity that he saw as 'manly'. Some sort of manual work would probably best achieve this, although Mr Wrigley's weak right hand may restrict the choice.

Maintenance antidepressant drugs should probably be given for at least a year at full dose. The antipsychotic medication should be gradually withdrawn once the depressive episode and psychotic features have resolved. Outpatient and community care follow-up should be offered for at least as long as this, and the GP encouraged to refer Mr Wrigley back at an early stage if he should subsequently relapse. Mr and Mrs Wrigley should also be given the name of a contact person, including the consultant, to get in touch with directly if this occurs.

CEREBRAL INFARCTION

Neurological advice should be sought about the use of a long-term antithrombotic agent, such as aspirin. A physiotherapy and an occupational therapy programme should be devised to exercise his hand.

SUICIDE RISK

Despite the precautions already discussed, there is a risk that treatment of any relapse may be as delayed or as inadequate as the recent treatment. The best safeguard against this is that someone who has seen him when he was severely depressed and who has also established a relationship of trust with him follow up Mr Wrigley.

*Prognosis*

Mr Wrigley is likely to recover from this episode but, as already mentioned, there is a significant risk of relapse whilst the circumstances that led to his depression continue. Mr Wrigley has also become further disabled as a result of his suicide attempt. He has noticeable scars on his wrists and throat, he has weakness of his right hand and he may have increased cognitive impairment. Should Mr Wrigley relapse, there is a high risk of a further suicide attempt, or successful suicide. The risk is increased by Mr Wrigley's tendency to dismiss the severity of his symptoms, and to mask his misery by superficial joviality.

The recurrence of depression will be made more likely if, as is possible, Mr Wrigley considers himself to blame for these disabilities. It would be considerably lessened if a suitable occupation could be found for him since

Mr Wrigley appears to have been free of depression, and to have coped well with adversity (such as the death of his mother), before his redundancy. Maintenance antidepressant treatment and the establishment of a rapid pathway to psychiatric consultation can also improve the prognosis, as would confidence in the psychiatrist and a greater readiness to consult him in the event of any deterioration.

## Further details

Mr Wrigley responded well to six twice-weekly ECT applications. He was discharged to a day hospital three weeks after beginning the course, apparently in normal spirits. His hand, although much improved, was still weak and Mr Wrigley blamed this on the cut on his wrist, saying, 'I shouldn't have done it, should I, doctor?' He had a rousing welcome home from his friends but his pleasure at returning to his social club was marred by the discovery that he could no longer join in the sing-songs. His voice since his tracheotomy was not strong enough to hold a sung note.

A case conference was called. Mrs Wrigley's medical notes were obtained, Mr Wrigley's notes studied afresh and Mr Wrigley interviewed again. The history then obtained was as follows.

### Further information

Mr Wrigley's father, Anthony, probably died of tuberculosis, leaving the family in very straitened circumstances. His mother had to get what work she could, which was sometimes only collecting rags for re-sale. The children occasionally went hungry and made use of the Church Army soup kitchen. There were four children: Anthony died of a brain tumour, Rosie died of an infection at the age of six months, Flo who had died recently, and Mr Wrigley was the youngest. Mr Wrigley's mother appeared to have inspired awe as well as love in Mr Wrigley. Despite their pinched circumstances Mr Wrigley remembered his childhood as very happy, and his family and their neighbours as being close and supportive. His sister and he continued to live in the same area after his mother died, 16 years before. About ten years before, they were dispersed by an urban renewal scheme and 'something was lost'. After his mother, Mr Wrigley was closest to Flo, who had stayed at home to look after their mother. After her death Flo married and she and her husband were in the habit of going with the Wrigleys every Sunday to put flowers on their mother's grave.

Mr Wrigley had been a lively boy whose main interest was sport. He played cricket for his school. He had little academic interest and left at 14 to work as a lathe operator.

As the result of a strike three years later he was made redundant and then worked for two years as a plumber's mate, until he was called up. Mr Wrigley served as a sapper in Cyprus and the UK during his national service. He was never promoted and had two periods in a military prison for drunkenness. He resented the pay he received, feeling that he was unable to provide as much for his mother as he wanted. In 1951 his brother was injured in an industrial accident and was retired on health grounds. He subsequently developed a brain tumour and died. The news reached Mr Wrigley whilst he was in hospital for treatment of dysentery. He requested compassionate leave, but this was turned down. He assumed that the accident had caused the tumour and felt incensed that his brother's employers paid no compensation to his mother. His reaction to the news may have prolonged his stay in hospital, although it was not clear whether he was depressed or simply angry.

Mr Wrigley then had various jobs in the building trade and two long periods as a labourer. The second job, with the Water Board, paid very well because it involved him in emergency work at night and weekends for which he received 'call-out' rates. He lost this job because he stole some lead piping belonging to his employers. He was charged for this and received a six-month prison sentence, suspended for two years. He had since frequently ruminated about the 'stupidity' of this theft, which was an impulsive one, committed, he said, 'only to help a mate'. Mr Wrigley's last job, with the hospital, came to an end when he had his first stroke. He was on sick leave for about six weeks and was then examined by a doctor acting on behalf of his employers, who recommended retirement on medical grounds. Mr Wrigley said they had treated him 'generously', because he received a lump sum and a small pension.

Mr Wrigley went out with his first girlfriend at the age of 16, but had no serious girlfriend until he met his wife at a dance after he began working. They married within a year and went to live with his mother. There were often rows about money at the beginning. Mr Wrigley liked to gamble at greyhound races and this prevented them from saving for a house. His mother eventually stepped in with an ultimatum – he 'either stopped or got out'. Since then he gambled much less, but still did so, usually on horseracing. Their son was born a year after they were married. His daughter was 'a mistake'. Although neither Mr nor Mrs Wrigley had wanted further children, Mr Wrigley assured the interviewer that he loved her, now, quite as much as his son.

Mrs Wrigley worked as a cleaner until about three years ago, when she developed asthma, and had not worked since. She had two recent episodes of illness, to be described later. One involved weight loss. Mrs Wrigley was strikingly thin even after treatment. Her usual weight was 80lbs and her height just under 5 feet. It was difficult to assess how husband and wife felt about each other. Mrs Wrigley only spoke about her concern in a veiled way; for example, 'I knew that he wasn't right when he'd apologize when I shouted at him instead of shouting back.'

When well Mr Wrigley spent three or four weekday evenings at the pub, sometimes with his wife, and regularly went to the British Legion with her on Saturdays. This was the most enjoyable part of his week. He drank 3–4 pints of bitter whenever he went out, and the occasional half a pint at home on other evenings. They lived in a rented, semi-detached, three-bedroom house with a pleasant garden. Mr Wrigley enjoyed doing odd jobs in both house and garden, but he was happiest in company. His wife described him as a 'man's man'.

Mr Wrigley's first stroke occurred when he was getting undressed. His right side began to shake and then became stiff. This worsened over several hours and he also developed slurred speech and a droop of the right side of his face. The facial palsy and dysarthria disappeared within a few days but a mild right hemiparesis was still present when he was examined by his GP eight months later, shortly after his second stroke. On this occasion he felt his left arm and leg become cold and weak and then felt himself falling to the left. For two weeks following this Mr Wrigley's gait was unsteady. He then developed shaking of his right side, which was worse in the morning. Retrospectively this was presumed due to anxiety, because it was at that time that his family noted a change in his mood. Mr Wrigley was referred to a neurologist for his shakiness. He was seen once, when early clubbing, minimal unsteadiness and a high erythrocyte sedimentation rate (ESR) were noted. He was then discharged.

Mrs Wrigley became ill herself in the meanwhile with what she now referred to as 'a depression'. She described herself as 'doing nothing and eating nothing' and just 'flopping in a chair'. This was attributed to 'over-stimulation' by her adrenergic inhalants.

The situation at home became worse. Mr Wrigley was prescribed benzodiazepines by his GP and was told to stop drinking. This resulted in his not going to the pub and losing contact with his friends. He began to go for long, lonely walks. His sister, Flo, had a stroke and this was found to be due to a cerebral metastasis. Mrs Wrigley kept his sister's illness from her husband for fear that he would think he had cancer too, but when she died he was 'too numb' to feel her death very strongly.

Eight months before admission Mr Wrigley was again referred to a neurologist with 'nervousness, shaking, poor appetite and inability to concentrate'. The neurologist noted that he was markedly depressed and had a classical anxiety tremor. He also noted increased tone and brisk reflexes in all four limbs, more on the left than the right, clonus of his left ankle and a 'probably extensor' left plantar reflex. A diagnosis of 'brain-stem ischaemia/infarction' was made and Mr Wrigley was put on the waiting list for further investigation in hospital.

The Saturday after this, Mr Wrigley suddenly shouted 'I can't stand any more of this' and ran into the kitchen. His sister in law ran after him and restrained him from pushing a carving knife into his abdomen. The blade had already penetrated a jumper and shirt and his skin. Mr Wrigley broke down after this, sobbing 'I'm sorry, I'm sorry', as already described.

Mr Wrigley was admitted to hospital three weeks later and Mrs Wrigley was admitted shortly after for investigation of weight loss. The arch aortogram was performed at this time and the MRI scan was later performed in outpatients with the results already described.

No physical explanation was found for Mrs Wrigley's weight loss, which was attributed to the 'stress of living with her husband'. (Her physician later commented in a letter to the GP that it was perhaps for the best that Mr Wrigley had cut his throat because 'at least now he will be getting treatment'.) She saw a psychiatrist who advised her 'to socialize more'. When she returned home, she found her husband's mood had deteriorated further. He roamed the house at night, banged the wall with his fists and avoided contact with family and friends. She tried to persuade her GP to refer him to a psychiatrist but he was reluctant to do so. The neurological SHO was also concerned about *his* weight loss and ordered an ultrasound scan of his liver and a barium enema, both of which were found to be normal. Six weeks later the consultant reviewed him in the clinic. He told Mr Wrigley that he had vertebro-basilar insufficiency, that the cause had been found and was under control, but that they had 'drawn a blank' about his weight loss. He recommended referral to a general physician. Mr Wrigley's symptoms did not change markedly between this time and his referral to the psychiatric clinic. He did not know what to do with himself and went for long walks or paced the floor. He visited his club very occasionally, but did not enjoy it. He avoided meeting people and he slept less and less.

On the day of his suicide attempt Mr Wrigley got up, as usual, at 6.30 a.m. as he would have done if he had been working. He had been awake but lying in bed for some hours before this, but had no particular thoughts of suicide. He went downstairs and heard the men next door and across the road going to work. He suddenly thought, 'What's the point?' He had a safety razor blade in his hand and he cut repeatedly into his left wrist with it. Thinking 'I might as well finish the job off', he transferred the blade to his left hand and cut his right wrist, and then, with the blade in his right hand, cut his throat. He felt heavy, and then cold, and remembered no more until he was in hospital. From his wife's account it appears that his daughter, who had to get up unusually early, went down a few minutes later and found her father jammed behind the toilet door. Neither she nor her mother had any intimation of what he had in his hand.

## Comments

The fresh history brought to light many details of the development of Mr Wrigley's illness, his personality and his background. Some missing information has been obtained; for example, he had another sibling who had died, Tracey was unplanned and he had been convicted of theft. Inaccuracies have also been corrected; in particular, the timing of his redundancy in relation to his illness. Even more important, a more secure and personal relationship with the psychiatrist has been established.

The events of Mr Wrigley's life now make sense because they are located in a personal context. Mr Wrigley's impulsive and nearly catastrophic suicide attempt can now be seen to be of a piece with his gambling and his impulsive theft; the anger motivating it can be seen to have been foreshadowed by his anger with the Army's refusal of compassionate leave to him and compensation for his mother, following his brother's death.

It might be argued that in a busy clinic, or in an examination, such detail cannot be obtained in one interview. Whilst this is true, we would argue that it is therefore necessary to spread the history-taking process over a number of interviews, which may include the period of illness and convalescence. One can only get to know a person, his or her family and social context over a period of time. It is when mutual trust has developed that people will reveal more about themselves. Only in this way can 'an ear' for expectable developments in a history be acquired. Once a psychiatrist's ear becomes attuned, understandable narratives can be obtained from much briefer interviews.

# Chapter 4

# *An Overdose*

## *Mary Brown*

## Presenting complaint

The duty psychiatrist was asked to see Mary who had been admitted to the Observation Ward following an overdose two days previously. This was described in the notes as an 'impulsive overdose' which followed a series of rows with her boyfriend. When she saw the psychiatrist, Mary said that she felt 'very confused' about the situation she was in and wanted to 'hear someone else's point of view'. She then gave the following account of the circumstances surrounding her overdose.

It followed one of her frequent rows with her boyfriend, Cyril. They went out for a walk and returned to his house to have sexual intercourse. Afterwards, he began to question her about her previous boyfriends and said he didn't trust her to be faithful. She then challenged him about his previous girlfriends and this developed into an argument. He then 'smacked me around the face and walked out of the room'. She said that she then felt 'frustrated and helpless' and picked up a bottle of aspirins which she kept under her pillow to treat headaches. She took all the aspirins in the bottle (about 45) because she 'just wanted to get out of this awful situation'. At that moment she believed she would have taken even more tablets if they had been available, although she generally had considerable difficulty swallowing even one. About half an hour later she began to feel sick and generally unwell. She then panicked and ran out to tell Cyril, who was downstairs. He tried to make her vomit by putting his fingers down her throat, but this failed and he called an ambulance that took her to the Casualty Department. After her stomach was washed out, Cyril continued to berate her about her previous affairs and she felt 'very relieved to be admitted to hospital'.

## Family history

Mary was adopted within a few months of her birth. Her adoptive mother was now 55 and managed a hairdressing salon. Mary said she 'switched between loving and hating her'. She generally found it easy to discuss problems with her, but her mother strongly disapproved of Cyril and they therefore avoided talking about him. Her adoptive father was 55 and managed an advertising agency. His physical health had deteriorated over the last 18 months during which time he had suffered several minor strokes. According to Mary, this meant that he was unable to maintain responsibility for his business and his partners had been forced to take over more of its active management. Apparently, he was unaware of this. She said that they got on 'quite well', but she found him difficult to talk to because he always saw things in 'black and white' terms.

She had a 19-year-old adoptive brother, John, and described their relationship as 'wonderful'. He was extremely intelligent and did well at school. She said that her parents approved of his friends and she thought that he was allowed far more freedom than her. Her adoptive mother had a stillbirth before she and John were adopted.

Mary said she was told nothing about her birth mother, but from conversations she overheard she believed that she was a French au pair who worked in Wales and became pregnant after an affair with a married man. When asked directly she said that she bore little resemblance to either of her adoptive parents, although she did look like John.

## Personal history

Mary was brought up in Liverpool and remembered her childhood as 'extremely happy'. She felt that knowing about her adoption from an early age never spoiled her relationship with her parents, and she had always called them 'Mum' and 'Dad'. She felt grateful to them for being so 'honest' and 'open' about this because it made their relationship more 'adult'. As far as she was concerned, the fact that she was physically dissimilar to both of them had never been a problem. The family were always very comfortably off. She had nice clothes and enjoyable holidays (frequently taken abroad) and they lived in a large, comfortable house.

She attended a local school from the age of four, which she described as 'enjoyable' and where she made many friends. Initially, she did quite well at school, became increasingly disinterested in her studies and was often told off by her teachers for talking in class. Eventually, she came to dislike it, and said, 'I do not think I would have liked any school I would have attended.' When she was 16 she passed 3 GCSEs, but felt she should have passed all the 6 subjects that she took. Although she had many friends at school, most of them lived a considerable distance away and she did not see them outside school hours. On occasions, she truanted with friends, but this was never discovered and she never came into serious conflict with her teachers.

After her examinations she left school and found herself a job as a beauty consultant, which she kept for six weeks. She got on badly with her supervisor and left to join a beauty consultant agency as a 'temp'. However, there was insufficient work and she left after four months. Following several months' unemployment she found herself another job as a receptionist for a voluntary organization, which she left after two weeks because she found it 'boring'. For the last 15 months she had been unemployed.

Her menarche occurred when she was 12. She did not start going out with boys until she was 15, when she had her first sexual relationship. This took place with a man 25 years older, while on a family holiday abroad. She then had numerous, brief sexual relationships that she said were 'very enjoyable'. Six months previously she met her current boyfriend, Cyril, at a party given by some of her brother's friends, and had no other boyfriends since. Cyril was 20 years old, black, unemployed and came from a large, working-class family. Her parents completely disapproved of this relationship, mainly because of his colour. This caused frequent rows at home and she began to spend increasingly less time at home and more time with him. Eventually, her mother told her to leave home and she found herself a flat.

For the last three months she had lived with Cyril and his family in their house, and said she had no other friends apart from them. She described his family as 'very supportive and friendly, but not pushy'. Since they were both unemployed, they spent practically all their time together and had frequent sexual intercourse. However, Cyril continually brought up details of her previous relationships and continued to criticize her for these. On occasions he physically assaulted her, but she said he never seriously hurt her and as far as she was concerned their relationship recovered soon after these arguments. The rows became increasingly frequent and she began to feel increasingly hurt and upset about his continual demand that she promise to be faithful. It was following one of these arguments that she took her overdose.

## Past medical history

Six months previously Mary was treated for a gonococcal infection, which she had contracted from Cyril.

Two months before she suffered a severe attack of herpes genitalis that had only just cleared up.

She had no other serious medical illness but did describe recurrent attacks of 'headaches', which she described as 'tightness around my head'. They usually followed her arguments with Cyril and were relieved by taking aspirins, which she kept under her pillow.

## Past psychiatric history

Mary gave no history of any previous psychiatric illness.

## Previous personality

She said she had always been a friendly, outgoing person and did not think she had changed.

## Mental state examination

*Appearance and general behaviour*

Mary was an overweight, but attractive woman, who smiled frequently during the interview and conveyed a sense of flirtatiousness. She was relaxed and self-composed and had clearly taken some care about her appearance, since she wore smart clothes and was effectively made up.

*Speech*

She spoke clearly and fluently, with a Liverpudlian accent.

*Mood*

Mary looked miserable when she talked about her arguments with Cyril; however, this was not sustained. She smiled frequently and mostly appeared cheerful. She had no worries about her physical health, was not particularly bothered by her headaches and did not give the impression of being concerned about her femininity. Although she frequently said that she felt 'guilty' about her promiscuity and her current relationship with her family, she did not convey this with any intensity. She described her current difficulties as 'unresolvable', but presented this as an intriguing state of affairs rather than a problem that overwhelmed her. She had never thought about taking an overdose before and 'certainly never' made any such threats to Cyril. She had no intention of killing herself at the time, but added, 'When you are feeling upset you don't care…' When asked directly she agreed that she had felt angry, but mainly upset. Following the overdose she became very frightened that she might die and was relieved to have obtained such speedy assistance. She now felt that it was 'a very silly thing to have done', but that it had at least forced a confrontation between Cyril and herself, and that this would be useful. However, she did not see it becoming a means of getting her own way in the future and she said she would never take an overdose again.

## Thought content

Mary talked a great deal about her intense feelings for Cyril. She said that she found him physically attractive and sexually satisfying and felt that he often showed considerable sympathy for the difficulties she experienced with her family. She also found his family relaxed, warm and friendly and felt that they had accepted and welcomed her. On the other hand, she found his continual cross-questioning about her previous relationships exhausting and frustrating and she was beginning to feel at a loss as to how she would ever be able to reassure him satisfactorily. She then said, 'I often feel I would be unable to reassure myself about this too.' She also felt that Cyril was very unreasonable to insist on her faithfulness when he continued to be promiscuous. As far as she was concerned she loved him, but 'I can't live with him and I can't live without him'.

She frequently called herself 'a slag' and said she understood why Cyril mistrusted her and continually sought reassurance. On the other hand, she now believed 'this is all behind me' and felt frustrated at having to repeatedly 'go over the past'. She felt certain she had changed and was fed up with being reminded about her previous relationships. When asked directly about these relationships she said that she had enjoyed the sexual side, but never really became emotionally involved with anyone before Cyril.

Mary expressed considerable curiosity about her birth mother and said that she hoped to find out more about her. She described how she had contacted Somerset House to obtain a copy of her birth certificate but was informed that this would not be made available until she was 18. She worried that her adoptive mother would get upset if she found out about this.

Mary frequently said how worried she felt about the situation at home. Looking after her adoptive father was increasingly difficult and she felt that she should have spent more time at home helping. She said that she felt irresponsible for leaving her parents to sort out these problems themselves and giving them extra worries about herself. However, she also said that there was no practical help she could offer at home anyway.

It was noticeable how frequently Mary said that she appreciated her family's care and concern for her, and also pointed out how she understood the difficulties they might have faced in bringing her up. However, she was never specific about these 'difficulties' and when asked directly about them she rejected the suggestion that they might have anything to do with her having been adopted.

She made it clear on several occasions that she did not want anyone in her family to be informed of her current situation.

*Abnormal beliefs and interpretations of events*
None were elicited.

*Abnormal experiences*
None were elicited.

*Cognitive state*
This was not formally tested, but Mary appeared well orientated in time and space and of above average intelligence.

*Self-appraisal*
Mary did not think that she was suffering from a psychiatric illness, but saw her overdose as a direct consequence of her argument with Cyril. She did not think it was a serious suicide attempt, but a way of getting herself out of an awkward situation. She thought that having taken the overdose 'things will probably settle down'.

## Physical examination

The physician had performed a thorough physical examination and nothing abnormal was found. Investigations showed that her serum salicylate level never reached a dangerous level and dropped to zero by the time she was examined by the psychiatrist.

## Ward observations

The nurses described Mary as a 'normal, cheerful girl' who talked freely and openly with them and the other patients on the ward. She was helping the elderly ladies there, by making cups of tea. She never cried and appeared to be sleeping and eating well. Her boyfriend had turned up on two occasions and they seemed to get on quite amicably.

## Preliminary assessment

Mary Brown is a 17-year-old adopted girl who has taken an overdose following an argument with her boyfriend.

Young females who have taken an overdose are unlikely either to have a persistent psychiatric disorder or to attend any follow-up appointment. As a result of this and other pressures, such as the general workload, psychiatrists generally set out to exclude a serious psychiatric disorder and avoid making management plans based upon a detailed evaluation of the individual's requirements. This may be justified on the grounds of expediency. However, it is not an approach that can generally be recommended and the wider issues in this case will therefore be considered.

### Diagnosis

Some of Mary's symptoms could be seen as manifestations of a depressive illness. On several occasions she said how 'guilty' she felt about both her previous sexual promiscuity and neglecting her family. She also denigrated herself by referring to herself as a 'slag'. However, these feelings were not conveyed with a morbid intensity and did not contain a hopeless quality. In fact, she appeared to accept them as a rather temporary state of affairs for which she did not feel totally responsible. Her feeling that she had no contribution to make to her family's welfare seemed to be less important than her relationship with Cyril, and although she regretted her past promiscuity she also said that she wanted Cyril to stop pestering her about it. Essentially, her feelings of 'guilt' appear to reflect a realistic discomfort with her current circumstances and a wish for the situation to be changed, rather than an unremitting, deep discontent with herself, over which she has no control.

There are no other features that might support a diagnosis of depression. She appeared cheerful, described no alteration in her sleep pattern and did not report any changes in her mood. This inference is supported by the nurses' observations of her behaviour. However, the information available does suggest that she had serious problems in establishing and maintaining interpersonal relationships. She has never had any long-standing, close friendship or childhood friend. Although her explanation for this was that she lived too far away from school, this does not explain why she was unable to make friends closer to her home. Her main relationships were with men, were brief, and seem to have been based predominantly on sexual attraction. Her longest sustained relationship, with Cyril, has the additional disturbing feature of frequent rows, occasionally developing into physical conflict.

Mary's school record suggests that she under-achieved and there is a suspicion that she had difficulties with her teachers as well as with her peers. Her work record reinforces the likelihood that she has problems with authority. According to her she had less difficulty obtaining employment than in holding down a job for any length of time. Although she gave 'boredom' as her reason for leaving, on at least one occasion she admitted to not getting on well with her employer.

Finally, although she avoided going into detail, she conveyed the impression that she had long-standing problems with her family. She had considerable conflict with them over Cyril and was forced to leave home on account of this. She implied that she found her brother more favoured by her parents, even though she said that they had a 'wonderful' relationship. Furthermore, the fact that she so strenuously attempted to understand why her parents might have had problems with her supports the belief that there were difficulties. This is reinforced by the importance she places upon Cyril's family's attitude towards her, which she described as 'warm and caring'. However, she steadfastly resisted being explicit about these issues.

Examination of her mental state also revealed several noteworthy features. In particular, she maintained a cheerful, relaxed posture in spite of her insistence that she was in an awful situation from which she felt she could not escape. This suggests quite marked dissociation of affect. She also appeared to obtain considerable gratification from discussing her problems while expressing the belief that she would have to sort them out herself. Finally, the psychiatrist was struck by the inconsistency between her manner, which he noted as 'charming' and which appeared inconsistent with the situation she was describing, and by the element of flirtatiousness in her behaviour. One effect of this was that he did not pursue her statements thoroughly. For example, he did not clarify whether the aspirins she kept under her pillow for 'headaches' reflected a long-standing preoccupation with self-harm.

In summary, Mary has had few close emotional relationships, apart from with her family and with Cyril, and these have been coloured by conflict. Her other relationships sound rather shallow, and she seems to have had particular difficulty in accepting control from authority. She also showed possible dissociation of affect and a seeming gratification from being in impossible situations. Furthermore, she presented herself in a way that made it very difficult to challenge or clarify important issues that emerged. Many of these characteristics can be observed at some time in most people, particularly when they are placed under stress. However, in Mary's case they were all present together and significantly coloured her behaviour, particularly in the context of her recent overdose.

Psychiatrists try to avoid making a diagnosis of personality disorder in younger people, because it implies that the problem is firmly established. Adolescence and early adulthood are often coloured by emotional turmoil, which settles down with maturity. Nevertheless this possibility needs to be considered. In Mary's case the features are compatible with a diagnosis of either a histrionic personality disorder or an acute adjustment reaction. The former is supported by the suggestion that these elements have coloured Mary's relationships since childhood and are now an established part of her character structure. However, it is also possible that although these elements are present, they contribute less significantly to her character and have been exaggerated by her current predicament. If the emphasis is placed on the significance of stress rather than her personality, then the diagnosis of acute adjustment reaction becomes more likely.

The distinction between these diagnoses is not always clear-cut and frequently depends upon evaluation of outcome. Furthermore, all the information has been provided by Mary and it requires independent confirmation to support one of these diagnoses. Suspicion remains, however, that the disturbances described are sufficiently ingrained to be considered a manifestation of a histrionic personality disorder.

## Aetiology

Mary has recently been subjected to several stressful factors that could have contributed to her overdose. Her adopted father is becoming physically and intellectually incapacitated as a result of several 'strokes'. His deterioration and the risk of further, possibly fatal, episodes would make Mary very vulnerable to an emotional disturbance. Although the time relationship between Mary's disorder and her adoptive father's illness has not been established, her account suggests that his deterioration may also have been associated with her leaving home.

Mary also described an episode of venereal disease. This might not only have been an upsetting experience, but the fact that herpes genitalis can be very painful could also have made it an additional provocative factor.

Her conflictual relationship with Cyril is also likely to have made Mary vulnerable to taking an overdose and their recent row seems to have been the most immediate trigger. However, she has never taken an overdose before, in spite of many previous fights, and it is unclear whether this row differed in some way from the others or whether it was the last of an accumulation of pressures.

She has also talked openly about her wish to trace her birth mother and she will soon be entitled to do this. Anxieties associated with this possibility may also have contributed to her stress at this time.

Although these factors explain why Mary was at risk of taking an overdose at this particular time, her personality is likely to have made her particularly vulnerable. It would not have been surprising if Mary's adoption had affected her personality development and her relationships with her adoptive family. The fact that she is so emphatic about rejecting this possibility strongly suggest 'denial'. She insisted, 'It has never been a problem.' She frequently said how 'grateful' she felt to her parents, because they were always so 'open' about her adoption. She said that she appreciated this and valued their care and attention, although she clearly felt that they favoured her brother. Furthermore, her statement that relationships at home were 'wonderful' was inconsistent with her mother's insistence that she leave.

It is possible that Mary's adoption was not as smooth as she described. Her account, particularly with its inconsistencies, might reflect that she did not always feel comfortable with, or accepted and loved by, her adoptive family and was uncertain about her true identity. This view is reinforced by the importance Mary has invested in her relationship with Cyril and his family.

Mary's romanticized account of her birth mother and the stereotyped description she gave of her adoptive parents suggests that she has not developed a clear sense of her own identity. This also colours her relationship with Cyril: 'I can't live with him and I can't live without him.'

The uncertainty about her background and her difficulty in believing that her adoptive family accepted her would have made it difficult for her to find an acceptable model with whom to identify during her development, and from whom she could learn to cope with stressful situations. These factors would also account for the fact that Mary seems to dissociate her feelings and present a rather 'novelettish' account of her history, which might seem to her to be more attractive than the uncertain situation that really exists.

Mary's vulnerability to stress may also have made her more liable to encounter situations in which she is likely to become stressed. An example of this is her conflictual relationship with Cyril. She seems to have managed her own insecurity by living with someone who is equally insecure. The fact that Cyril was unemployed and extremely jealous was balanced by his apparent capacity to demonstrate affection and the fact that he came from a family she perceived as warm and close.

*Further information*

Although psychiatrists may make decisions based upon one interview, this is generally an unsatisfactory course of action to follow and it is important to try to obtain information from independent sources. One reason, in Mary's case, is that she might not have given an entirely honest account of herself. The likelihood that she is distorting the truth is reinforced by the melodramatic flavour of her story. If this is so it would alter both the diagnostic and aetiological possibilities.

The most obvious sources of information are Mary's adoptive parents and Cyril. Her adoptive family should be asked to describe her early development, in particular whether she has always been a disobedient child who was difficult to control. They could confirm whether such traits affected her education and resulted in poor school reports or truancy and if they thought this also contributed to her poor work record. They could also give more information concerning her adoption and how much of this was discussed with Mary. The details of Mary's adoptive father's illness should also be clarified, as should the impact of Mary's relationship with Cyril upon her family. An account should be obtained of her general relationships with a peer group and any suspicion that Mary abused drugs.

Cyril could also give his account of their relationship. In particular he could describe their rows in more detail and he could report whether Mary has threatened to take an overdose in the past, or whether he was surprised by this action. It would also be useful to know the extent to which his family welcomed Mary.

While attempting to verify these details, the psychiatrist should also attempt to evaluate Mary's relationships with the informants. In particular, it might become apparent whether certain issues would benefit from joint counselling, which would depend on whether Mary intends to return home or to carry on living with Cyril. More complicated factors, such as her motivation for joint counselling, could also be assessed. For these reasons joint interviews should be encouraged.

*Management*

The main aim is to reduce the risk that Mary will take further, serious overdoses when she is placed under stress. This might be achieved by exploring ways in which she can be helped to become less vulnerable, by introducing her to less dangerous and more appropriate ways of communicating her distress, or by looking for particular areas of stress that might be effectively reduced. All of these approaches can be included within a counselling programme that could be undertaken individually or jointly with Mary's family and/or with Cyril. In this way particular areas of difficulty could be focused on, such as her rows with Cyril, her difficulty coping with her father's illness, or possible problems concerning her adoption. These alternatives all require her cooperation over an extended period of time and it is therefore necessary to encourage her to attend the Outpatient Department for follow-up and for her relatives and Cyril to be interviewed.

In order to achieve this, the psychiatrist will need to emphasize that he considers her situation to be serious, but that he thinks there are several ways in which he might be able to help her. It would probably also be helpful if he points out straight away to Mary that he does not think she has a psychiatric illness and that she will have to share the decisions regarding further treatment.

## Prognosis

Any prediction about the outcome of this episode, in particular Mary's risk of taking another overdose, can only be offered in the uncertainty that surrounds much of the information she has provided. Further details of her personality development, background and current situation may well affect the prognosis.

In spite of these reservations, most of the available information suggests that Mary has a high risk of further self-harm. She seems to have a personality that makes her vulnerable to stress, she has few friends, lacks internal resources and there is a suspicion that she has had difficulties with authority for some time. Furthermore, she is currently unemployed and has had numerous short-term relationships, both of which increase her vulnerability. Finally, her current relationship with Cyril involves a considerable amount of conflict and has already led to this hospital admission. If she returns to the same situation it seems likely that the stresses will continue.

## Further details

The psychiatrist who assessed Mary accepted her account. He formed the opinion that she had a personality disorder and had taken her overdose as a response to her argument with Cyril. He asked to speak to Cyril and her family, but she refused to let him. He then suggested that she attend the outpatients in order to discuss her problems further, but she declined this offer as well.

He then decided not to pressurize her any further because he thought she was determined not to attend for follow-up. He considered it more useful to acknowledge this and to suggest that if she were to change her mind he would be pleased to see her again. He also pointed out that she could contact her general practitioner if she felt a further crisis was developing and that this would be a better way of communicating her distress, than to acquire the habit of taking overdoses. Mary smiled and said, 'I have to sort out my problems for myself.' She said she had no intention of taking another overdose, but agreed to contact the psychiatrist if she changed her mind.

Following her discharge from hospital, the psychiatrist contacted her general practitioner, who had known Mary and her family for many years. He gave the following account of her background.

Mary was adopted within two weeks of her birth. The senior partner of the practice, who knew both Mary's birth mother and her adoptive family, arranged the adoption privately. Her current general practitioner had never met Mary's birth mother but knew that she came from a family with an infamous reputation within the local community. They lived in an extremely deprived area and had a reputation for conflict with the police over petty theft and alcoholism. Even within the local community they were considered particularly difficult and made more use of the social services department than other needy families. Mary's general practitioner remarked spontaneously upon the contrast between Mary's birth mother and her adoptive parents' social backgrounds. He confirmed that her adoptive parents were both successful, professional people, that Mr Brown was suffering from a severe pre-senile dementia and that he was now totally incapable of running his business independently. As a result the business was being wound down and this was causing his wife considerable strain, both emotional and financial.

Mary had been difficult from a very early age. As a small child her parents frequently complained about her naughtiness, which contrasted markedly with the docility of her adoptive brother. The general practitioner's daughter attended the same private school as Mary, where she had a reputation for being difficult, and was associated with a group of girls who were known for their persistent disobedience and lack of academic success. He also believed that there was an episode when she was involved in petty theft, but that her family hushed up the matter. She frequently ran away from home and three months ago she had left to live with an Afro-Caribbean boy, who was unknown to him.

The general practitioner was not surprised that Mary had taken an overdose in view of the problems he noted over the years in her relationships with her family and others.

The psychiatrist also contacted the Registrar for Births and Deaths to clarify the process whereby adoptive children are able to trace their birth parents. This confirmed Mary's account that adopted children without birth certificates are only able to obtain the appropriate records after they have reached 18 years of age. The psychiatrist also received an information pack, which explained the importance of counselling for children who pursue this aim.

## Reassessment

Mary's current social situation has been broadly confirmed, whereas the details of her adoptive family and previous personality are not wholly unsuspected. The reader should consider whether the psychiatrist would have been able to 'engage' her more successfully if he had obtained this information earlier.

### Diagnosis

The additional information makes much clearer the long-standing nature of Mary's problems. Her parents and her schoolteachers have always found her 'difficult'. There is also a suggestion that she has previously displayed antisocial tendencies, such as her possible involvement in theft. However, it is the fact that her behavioural problems have been present from a very early age and seem to have become established aspects of her personality that increase the likeliness of histrionic personality disorder.

## Aetiology

The fact that Mary was adopted also takes on increasing significance. It suggests how her personality development may have been affected, as well as why she has presented at this time.

It may appear strange that her personality resembled her birth mother's so closely in contrast to that of her adoptive parents. One possible explanation for this is that she was far more aware of her mother's character than she revealed and in some way identified with her. This awareness need not necessarily have been fully conscious and it is possible that her parents knew her birth mother's background and communicated this to her, in spite of efforts to protect her from this knowledge. Although Mary will probably have inherited some personality characteristics from her mother, it is unlikely that this explains such a complicated mixture of traits as Mary demonstrates.

As far as the timing of Mary's overdose is concerned, the approach of her eighteenth birthday means that she is now in a position to trace her birth mother. Given the clearer picture of her birth mother's background, the contrast between this and her stated expectation would be confronted, and would result in considerable and understandable distress.

Finally, the general practitioner has also confirmed that Mary's adoptive father is becoming increasingly incapacitated by a pre-senile dementia, which is causing considerable distress for his family. This stress appears to have been related to Mary leaving home as well as her recent overdose.

## Further information

It would be useful to know how aware Mary's adoptive family were of her background and the extent to which this had been overtly or covertly transmitted to her.

*Management*

The additional information suggests that if any further action can be taken it should be for Mary to obtain specific counselling focusing on her adoptive father's illness, and the circumstances of her birth family and her adoption. The main difficulty with this is that Mary has decided not to see the psychiatrist again and therefore the possibility of writing to her, offering such a course of action, should be considered.

It seems unlikely, given her previous history and the evidence from the interview, that she will accept such a course of action. On the other hand, although it may be more expedient not to contact her, it might be more productive to give her the opportunity of refusing a specific offer of help. An alternative approach would be to inform the general practitioner, who could refer her back later.

*Prognosis*

Mary remains at a high risk of taking further overdoses, whether she succeeds in tracing her mother or not. Her personality appears to be well established and she has shown considerable resistance to accepting offers of help.

## Postscript

The psychiatrist decided not to contact Mary again. However, he did contact her general practitioner six months later and established that neither he nor the hospital had received any information about subsequent overdoses.

Chapter 5

# Fear of Becoming Fat

## Jane Morgan

## Presenting complaint

Jane Morgan was a 17-year-old girl referred by her general practitioner to the psychiatric outpatient department because of severe weight loss and a dread of becoming fat.

One year earlier she had begun to diet with a group of girlfriends at the college she was attending. She weighed 8½ stones (54kg) then and was 5ft 4in tall. Jane's initial aim was to lose 'about half a stone' (3kg) and she was particularly keen to take some fat off her thighs. Within a few weeks the other girls started to give up their diets whereas Jane found that she was able to persist in eating less. She felt proud of this and decided to see how much more weight she could lose. Over the next six months she dropped to 6st 13lb (44kg). She then started eating even less and stopped her mother from cooking an evening meal for her. At this time she was eating only about 600 calories per day, with a typical evening meal consisting of 3 or 4 crisp breads, spread thinly with cucumber spread. Occasionally she would eat fish but only if it was grilled. As well as this she exercised vigorously in her room every evening.

Jane went on holiday with her mother to Spain in the summer when she weighed 6st 6lb (41kg). There she walked whenever possible and with the rest of the party contracted a gastrointestinal disorder which gave her diarrhoea. She was pleased about this and deliberately ate a lot of fruit to make it worse. It helped her to lose more weight and on her return from holiday she weighed 6st (38kg). Despite this she insisted on playing lacrosse with her club.

When her mother offered her food she became angry and stormed out of the room. When she did eat at home she frequently did so standing up and would immediately go out for a long walk. At this time Jane weighed herself six times every day and felt relieved when she noted a further loss of weight.

Two months before presentation to the psychiatric clinic, her mother finally coaxed Jane into going to see the family doctor. She weighed 5st 9lb (36kg) and was now too exhausted to play lacrosse. The doctor, however, was unable to persuade her to eat more and finally referred her to the psychiatrist.

During the last few months Jane had also become extremely fastidious about housework. She was almost continually tidying up and putting things away. She took over nearly all of the family cooking and prepared rich and elaborate dishes which she pressured her mother into consuming. She was preoccupied with the need not to waste food. She felt very active and alert and woke at 5 a.m. every day.

One month before her visit to the clinic her father returned from Los Angeles because of his concern about her condition. Her parents insisted that she stop work at this time.

It had been a struggle to get Jane to the clinic but she finally relented because 'my mother looked so miserable'.

## Family history

Jane's parents separated when she was 18 months old, and later divorced. Her father, aged 52, was an executive for an oil company and he now lived in Los Angeles. Jane described him as a 'fitness fanatic' who was always concerned about 'healthy living'. He was in the habit of jogging 3–4 miles every day and he had a particular loathing for 'fat' people. He was a man who read extensively and who always liked to be right in an argument. Everyone regarded him as a 'born leader' and he was energetic in pursuing his aims. Despite the divorce, Mr Morgan maintained regular contact with his family and visited them every year, usually bringing expensive presents for the children. Jane remembered that he always seemed to like having attractive women around him.

Jane's mother was 47 and until recently had been a housewife, financially supported by her ex-husband. She had six months previously become a registered child minder. Jane described her mother as someone who 'feels deeply but can't express her feelings to others'. In many respects she was the opposite of Jane's father, seeming to be unsure about herself and finding it difficult to make decisions. She was a deeply religious woman and her social activities were restricted to the Church. Her appearance was of little concern to her and despite being a little overweight, she had never attempted to diet.

Jane did not know why her parents had separated. She believed, however, that her mother still missed her father and she had never shown any interest in other men. She suspected that her father had many girl-friends. She said she had a good relationship with both of her parents. She felt particularly close to her mother and they spent much time together. She often felt intimidated by her father's overbearing personality, but felt excited when she knew he was due to visit.

Jane had one sister, Rachel, aged 21, who was a secretary and had left her mother's home to join her father in the USA six months earlier. Since the age of 18 she had 'itchy feet' and always wanted to travel. She had been to visit her father when he was stationed in New York and later in Los Angeles. She expressed dissatisfaction with home and complained that her mother and Jane were dull, wishing only to go to church. Jane described Rachel as 'practically like father – intelligent and outspoken'. The two sisters used to fight 'like cat and dog' but the relationship had improved recently. Rachel was a constant dieter. When she was 18 she lost quite a lot of weight but quickly put it on again. Jane often teased her about her diets in the past.

There was no family history of psychiatric or physical illness.

## Personal history

Jane was born in Dallas, Texas, where her father was working at the time. Her parents had lived there for six years having emigrated from England. In the first two years of Jane's life, her parents moved frequently, four times in the space of one year. When she was 18 months old her parents separated and for the next five years her father visited most Saturdays.

Despite her parents' problems, Jane described her early childhood as a happy one. She showed no behavioural problems.

When Jane was 7, her mother brought her and her sister to England, while her father remained in the USA. Jane remembered the return as a 'great adventure'. They lived with her grandmother for about a year and then moved into the house in which Jane and her mother still lived.

Jane enjoyed junior school, both in the USA and later in England. She made friends easily and was popular on her return because of the novelty of her American accent. She said she was not very bright at school and found it difficult to remember what she should have learnt. However, she excelled at sports and sang in the school choir. She left school at 16, with two GCSEs, having failed two others. She said she disliked it, as she had to travel long distances to get there. Eventually she passed the other two GCSEs in English and Religious Knowledge and also did a typing course. Her school experiences had made her feel 'definitely not academic'.

Immediately after leaving college Jane obtained a job as a secretary in a small frozen food firm, where she worked for a year up to the time of her presentation to hospital. She loved the work because it was varied and because the people were very kind to her. They had shown a lot of concern about her thinness but she was not irritated by this. Her boss told her father that he would keep the job open because she was a 'good little worker'.

Jane had her menarche at 15 years. This was later than her friends who had teased her for being a 'baby'. Her periods were regular until eight months previously, stopping when she weighed 7st 1lb (45kg).

Jane was not interested in boys. For her and her best friend 'lacrosse was our life'. Her friend, however, became engaged nine months previously and they now rarely saw each other. Her mother always put a 'damper' on her and boys. 'I was always Mum's girl.' Despite being asked out often at college, she had never had a boyfriend. She was taught at church that sex was sinful and disliked the idea of being fondled by boys. She also did not think she could get a steady boyfriend because she was not 'perfection'. She was scared of boys hurting her. When asked if she was sexually attracted to girls she indicated that this was a disgusting suggestion.

## Past medical history

Jane had suffered no serious illness in the past. However, when she was 15 she had a cosmetic operation to remove a birthmark on her forehead, having been very sensitive about this 'deformity' for some years. The result was not totally satisfactory to her and she ensured that her forehead was always covered by her hair.

## Previous personality

Jane had always been a 'sports fanatic'. She had been in many school teams and represented her county at lacrosse. She was also a very strong squash player, but recently lacked the energy to play. She was also very musical, played the piano and recorder, and was a good singer.

She found it easy to make friends and was generally a cheerful and popular girl with a sense of humour that was often complimented by others.

She had always been conscientious in her work and tended to live an orderly life. She liked fixed routines and felt uneasy if these were disturbed.

She attended church regularly with her mother but, although she was religious, she was not as devout as her mother. She did not smoke or drink alcohol and had never experimented with any illicit drugs.

## Mental state examination

*Appearance and general behaviour*

Jane was a wide-eyed, alert, emaciated girl who would obviously have been very attractive if she were not so thin. During the initial part of the interview she responded sullenly to questions but brightened up as it progressed. She made it clear that she was only there under duress and was only cooperating on account of her parents' wishes. 'I know I am worrying my parents half to death.'

### Speech

Jane gave a very articulate account of herself.

### Mood

She had been feeling depressed over the previous three months, and attributed this to her mother's 'unreasonable fussiness' about her eating. On occasions she had been tearful but denied any feelings of hopelessness about the future. 'If people would only leave me alone everything would be OK.' She expressed some guilt about the effect she had on her mother but the worst guilt was when she ate 'too much'. Her social life was now very poor: 'I don't feel like going out – if people ring I get Mum to answer and make up excuses. I just feel like hiding in a corner.' She had lost interest in singing in the church choir: 'I don't have the energy to sing any more.' She had difficulty with her sleep and woke at 5 a.m.: 'Sometimes it hurts when I roll over in bed.' However, she felt bright and active in the morning. She had never thought life was not worth living and had never contemplated suicide. She admitted that sometimes she got 'confused'. 'I get angry with myself and say, "What am I playing at?" But then I decide that I can cope all right.' Since her father's return she had felt better, 'We've had a good sing-song together.'

Although Jane denied any anxieties other than those surrounding eating, she was somewhat troubled by her 'obsession with housework and order. If something has been moved, I have to get up and put it back in its right place; or if something has been messed up, I have to clean it right away.' She recognized that this was silly but could not stop herself no matter how hard she tried. 'It's amazing because I used to be so untidy in the past.'

### Thought content

Jane insisted she was not thin. 'I feel as if I am 8 and a half stone. When I look in the mirror, I don't look thin.' She preferred her abdomen to be 'completely flat' and thought that her 'troublesome' thighs were now 'about right'. She liked seeing her hipbones through her flesh. Jane admitted to hunger at times now, but for most of the past year she said she had not felt hungry at all. She also confided in a dread of seeing a weight increase when she stood on her scales. She said that she ate 'lots' but that she avoided 'unnecessary' foods. These included 'self-indulgent' foods containing sugar and fats. If she ate more than was 'necessary' she felt extremely guilty. 'I feel that I am doing something wrong, something that I shouldn't be doing.'

Her intake of food was very meagre and identical each day – a 5oz tin of baked beans, one egg, and crisp breads with cucumber spread. She did not allow her mother to prepare it for her as 'she might try to cheat'. She carefully counted calories and aimed for 'well under 1000 per day'.

Other measures aimed at accelerating her weight loss, apart from exercising excessively, were denied. She had thought about inducing vomiting after eating but decided it was 'too disgusting'. She said she did not abuse laxatives.

Jane's main preoccupations were with food and weight. 'I guess it's on my mind nearly 100 per cent of the time – I think, "When will I have to eat next, what will I have?"'

*Abnormal beliefs and interpretations of events*
None were elicited apart from ideas related to her weight.

*Abnormal experiences*
None were elicited.

*Cognitive state*
She seemed a girl of average intelligence and there were no cognitive deficits on clinical testing.

*Self-appraisal*

By the end of the interview, Jane was beginning to admit that she was not completely well. She was becoming easily exhausted and had lost interest in her previous activities. She worried about the fine hair that had grown over her arms and neck. 'I know you think I've got the slimmer's disease; if I do then it's not a bad case though. I don't make myself vomit. I used to love food so much. I know I can eat and eat and eat.' When asked the highest weight she could tolerate, she replied, 'I don't know. I mightn't mind going up to 7 stones (45kg) – but definitely no higher.' Her response to whether she was concerned about her periods stopping was, 'I don't mind at all. It's convenient really. It's not like I am trying to have children, is it?' She ended the interview by saying: 'I feel like a hypocrite being here. I don't need anything.'

## Physical examination

Jane was emaciated and weighed 5st 5lb (34kg). Her blood pressure was 100/70, her pulse was 64, and her periphery was cyanosed. There was lanugo hair on her forearms, the nape of her neck and the sides of her face.

## Interview with informants

Mr and Mrs Morgan were seen together without Jane.

Mrs Morgan confirmed the details of the development of the illness as given by Jane. Both parents commented that Jane had changed dramatically over the past year. She used to be a popular, friendly, good-humoured girl who was always 'sensible and obedient' at home. She had always been sensitive about her appearance, particularly her thighs. Father said, however, that she had good reason to worry about her thighs as they were 'on the big side'. Mother disagreed.

Mr Morgan dominated most of the interview. Very distressing for him was Jane's 'lashing out'. 'She has said some very disturbing things to her mother and me, even hurtful things. Is it just the food deprivation?' One example of this was when she said angrily, 'Others have fathers but I don't.' She had never shown feelings like this before. Both parents expressed horror at Jane's weight loss and felt hopeless about their attempts to get her to eat more. They felt they had tried everything.

Mrs Morgan described Rachel's leaving home as 'the last straw'. The sisters had been close up till then, and when Rachel left, Jane's weight plummeted.

Both parents remarked on Jane's dependency since she started losing weight. Mother said she was at her side all day and would start crying if she decided to go somewhere alone. Father said that since his return Jane had clung to him as well; 'She lets me hug her now whereas she didn't before.'

Mr Morgan said that he would stay in England as long as necessary to organize Jane's treatment. Mrs Morgan responded to this by saying: 'Yes, but after that you'll go away again.' Mr Morgan then said he would spend all of his leave entitlement in England until Jane was well again.

As Jane's parents were leaving the room, Mr Morgan dropped back to have a private word with the doctor. He said he thought that one factor in her illness was her mother not wanting Jane to go out, because she was apparently unhappy being left alone at night. She had told him she wanted to be more independent, but felt she couldn't because she had to stay and look after mother. The tone of his voice when talking about his ex-wife was obviously critical.

## Preliminary assessment

Jane is a 17-year-old girl who presents with a one-year history of severe weight loss. Although the diagnosis of anorexia nervosa and its management by encouraging weight gain appear straightforward in Jane's case, the problem is to gain her cooperation with treatment. In order to do this the psychiatrist requires knowledge of the available treatment options, the likely outcome and, perhaps most important of all, the complex way in which a variety of factors have contributed to Jane's presentation at this time.

*Diagnosis*

The clinical picture is typical of anorexia nervosa according to both ICD10 and DSMIV (restricting subtype). She shows a purposive reduction in food intake, particularly of 'fattening' foods, aimed at reducing her weight. Jane's weight has fallen from 54kg to 34kg. She has also used other measures to accelerate her weight loss, especially excessive exercise and on one occasion deliberately exacerbated a bout of diarrhoea. She also has had secondary amenorrhoea for six months. Finally, she exhibits a characteristic psychopathology. This involves a morbid fear of fatness, a relentless pursuit of thinness, and a disturbance of her body image in which she denies abnormality in her size in the face of severe emaciation. Jane gives an unrealistically low weight for the highest target weight she is prepared to countenance reaching.

Jane is in the usual age group where anorexia arises and the history is fairly typical. There have been a number of other changes that are frequently seen in conjunction with this disorder. These include a loss of interest in previously enjoyed activities, social withdrawal, depressive feelings and some obsessional traits. There are no serious differential diagnoses in Jane's case. Organic causes for weight loss are not accompanied by the typical psychopathology evidenced by Jane. Although there were some depressive symptoms these are in part due to her state of self-starvation and they are not sufficient to make a primary diagnosis of a depressive illness. Guilt about eating, loss of interest, early morning waking and eventual exhaustion are very common in anorexia nervosa.

There is also the possibility that Jane has an obsessional disorder. Her premorbid personality had some obsessional features such as her liking for order and routine and these have been accentuated recently. Her need to constantly clear up has the hallmarks of an obsessional impulse, in that there was a subjective compulsion, which she attempted to resist, and which she recognized as being senseless. However, her drive to diet did not have these features. She made no attempt to resist it, nor did she regard it as silly. On the contrary, she valued it highly. It is not unusual for obsessional symptoms to develop in the course of anorexia nervosa and they usually improve with weight restoration. Depressive symptoms behave similarly.

The diagnosis of anorexia nervosa thus appears straightforward.

*Aetiology*

Anorexia nervosa usually develops after a period of 'normal' dieting. The more frequently dieting occurs in a particular population, the more cases of anorexia will develop. It is very high, for example, amongst ballet students.

Even before Jane developed her illness, she was sensitive about her appearance. This is suggested by her cosmetic operation on her forehead and her concern about her thighs. Her father might have reinforced this by his apparent acceptance that Jane's thighs were too large, and in his pleasure, at least as perceived by Jane, in being surrounded by attractive and healthy women. These considerations help us to understand why both Jane and Rachel dieted seriously, but not why Jane developed anorexia nervosa, a condition that has made her both unattractive and unhealthy. Another factor, which might have assisted Jane in losing a lot of weight initially, was her concern with control. She is conscientious, hard-working and self-controlled, and probably brought these qualities to bear on her attempt at weight reduction. It may be that in finding other areas of her life difficult to control, especially interpersonal relationships with her parents and with boys (discussed below), she invested more of her energies in an area which she could control more readily, her body shape. This could have been facilitated by a relative insensitivity to internal cues, a secondary effect of sustained dietary restriction or, as has been suggested by some authorities, based upon a 'constitutional' predisposing factor to anorexia nervosa.

There are a variety of possible perpetuating factors for Jane's illness. Jane's distortion of body image, where she sees herself as being of normal weight, or even fat, when she is emaciated, provides the basis of a vicious cycle. Many patients with anorexia nervosa over-estimate their body size to a greater extent when they are thin and their perceptions become more accurate as they move closer to their healthy weight.

Other possible effects of the starvation itself need also to be considered. These include irritability, depression, preoccupation with food and impaired concentration. As a consequence of these, Jane may feel even less able to cope with her problems, which may in turn intensify her need to remain 'in control' of her diet.

Jane's history suggests some rivalry between her and her sister. Since Rachel has not been successful in maintaining a consistent weight reduction whereas Jane has, she may be loathe to relinquish her superiority in this regard.

Although Jane has been popular with her friends and has managed to do well at her work, she seems to have some difficulty in coping with her sexual feelings and with boys. She sees sex as 'sinful', fears being fondled, never accepts invitations from boys to go out and is pleased that her periods stopped. Anorexia nervosa may have helped her to cope with this problem by making her look and feel more like a prepubertal girl and less like a sexually mature young woman. Her self-starvation serves to flatten her feminine curves, to stop her periods and to extinguish sexual thoughts and feelings. It could be seen as having provided a welcome relief from these issues.

The illness has also ended Jane's moves to establish independence from her mother. She has become clinging, like a small child. Following Rachel's departure from home, Jane's weight fell dramatically. Jane has a very close relationship with her mother and were she to leave home as well then both would be likely to experience a great sense of loss. Mother would then be left alone without anyone to support her. She must have invested much in her children following her separation from Mr Morgan. The pain of such a separation is avoided by Jane's illness. In fact, Jane has become again a dependent little girl who needs to be looked after, even fed. In this context, it may be significant that Mrs Morgan has recently become a child minder. This may be the role in which she feels most comfortable. Rachel's departure to join Mr Morgan may have generated fears in Mrs Morgan that Jane will do the same, which would add to her sense of loss. Father's comment to the doctor that Mrs Morgan fears being left alone might have a strong element of truth.

Mr Morgan has maintained a close contact with his family despite 15 years of separation. From both Mrs Morgan's comments to her husband during their interview with the doctor, as well as Jane's account, it seems likely that she would like her ex-husband to return. Jane's illness has heightened his involvement with the family and it may be perpetuated, in part, by serving to reconstitute the family around the crisis it engendered.

The discussion above suggests that a variety of influences may be at work in shaping Jane's illness. These include factors understandable at physiological, psychological, interpersonal and socio-cultural levels.

## Further information

Further investigations aimed at evaluating Jane's physical status should be undertaken. It is important to assess her serum electrolytes since a hypokalaemic alkalosis would suggest that she is secretly inducing vomiting. A number of abnormalities might be revealed by other tests, such as a full blood count and liver function, but these are of uncertain significance in anorexia nervosa seeming to be the result of self-starvation. LH (luteinizing hormone), FSH (follicle-stimulating hormone) and oestrogen assays will be low for similar reasons, but they are not essential investigations.

More important, from the point of view of management, will be a fuller assessment of the psychological and family factors discussed under aetiology. The importance of the observations already made can be further supported or rejected following more interviews with Jane and with her family.

## Management

In all patients with anorexia nervosa the essential short-term goal is to restore weight and the longer-term goal is to maintain it at a healthy level. Until the patient is restored to a reasonable weight psychotherapeutic measures are generally not effective. This is because the consequences that the patient fears, and which need to be tackled in treatment, are avoided and less clearly manifest when she is emaciated.

Left to her own devices, Jane would not be expected to gain a substantial amount of weight. It might be possible for her mother, with a great deal of support from the doctor, to put pressure on Jane to eat more. However, the simplest and most certain means of ensuring weight gain is by admission to hospital, where Jane can be supervised and supported by nursing and medical staff. The initial obstacle to treating Jane will probably be to get her to accept admission.

Although she has not accepted that she is emaciated and that she needs help, her statements during the interview suggested some uncertainty about this. She admitted to a number of distressing feelings and the doctor can build on these to gain her cooperation. Her parents will probably also support putting pressure on her to accept admission. The psychiatrist will need to be firm and insistent that this is the proper course to take. At the same time the psychiatrist will need to make it clear to Jane that although her fears of weight gain are understood, admission will be essential if she is to be helped with some of the underlying problems that trouble her. Several interviews may be necessary to persuade her to accept admission. Although resort to admission under compulsory order might need to be considered, as Jane's condition is potentially life threatening, in practice this rarely proves necessary.

The inpatient phase of treatment will be directed to restoring Jane to a healthy weight, in the region of her premorbid weight of 54kg. It requires skilled nursing care to overcome her resistance to weight gain and to achieve this. She will need a nurse to supervise her meals and be with her for most of the day. Success will be most likely with nurses who understand the condition well and are able to demonstrate a combination of firmness and sympathy.

Jane needs to gain about 20kg and this will require about two months in hospital. When she nears her healthy weight she will be given increasing opportunities to eat unsupervised and she will eventually have weekends at home. A strict 'behavioural' regime is not necessary. Nor, given experienced nursing, is tube feeding.

During the course of her stay in hospital further meetings with her and her family will be aimed at gaining a better understanding of her difficulties, and to plan management following her discharge, in the light of this. She will probably need follow-up treatment as an outpatient for at least a year. The potential benefits of individual psychotherapy or family therapy will need to be assessed. The follow-up treatment will be directed at helping Jane to maintain her weight and to help her resolve those problems which have been previously 'solved' by self-starvation.

*Prognosis*

In the short term the prognosis for weight gain is good. It is likely that Jane will eventually accept admission to hospital and in hospital she will be restored to a near healthy weight. It is also likely that her attitude to her body and her depressive feelings will improve. The specific effects of malnutrition on Jane's physical and mental state is important and, when reversed, is likely to result in a major improvement. Although she is likely to restart menstruation after she achieves her expected weight, this may be delayed for a number of months and does not seem to affect the outcome.

The long-term prognosis is more difficult to assess. A number of factors in Jane's case suggest a good prognosis: the relatively short history of about one year (a 'long history' in this condition would be regarded as three years or more); the early age of onset; her good premorbid social adjustment in terms of interpersonal relationships and work, which usually has a particularly important bearing on the eventual outcome; and finally, the absence of bulimic episodes and self-induced vomiting.

Overall, the known prognostic features for this condition all point to an eventual recovery in Jane's case.

## Further details

Jane accepted admission to hospital after the first interview, to give her 'parents a rest'. She was in fact admitted to a unit that specializes in the treatment of anorexia nervosa and there were no particular difficulties in ensuring that she reached 54kg. She was in hospital for ten weeks altogether, but lost some weight during two weekends at home. Her weight on discharge was 51kg. All physical investigations were normal, apart from the expected low LH, FSH and oestrogen levels. At the time of her discharge Jane said that she felt 'a lot healthier' and more cheerful. She admitted, however, that she felt 'fat' at 51kg and that she would like 'to lose about half a stone' (3kg).

During her stay in hospital Jane was seen regularly on an individual basis. Her displeasure with her weight gain was very evident as was her reluctance to talk about other aspects of her life. Sullen nods were a frequent response to questions put to her. Mr Morgan returned to the USA two weeks after Jane's admission to hospital and he was due to come back to England for two weeks three months later. Sessions with Jane's mother supported the view that there was a marked interdependence between them and that this was an important contributing factor to Jane's illness. Their relationship seemed to require Jane to be a 'little girl'.

In view of the prominent family factors and of Jane's reluctance to engage in individual therapy, it was decided that following discharge Jane would be seen together with her mother, with her father and Rachel attending when they were in England.

In the first three months of follow-up treatment the hypothesis that Jane's symptoms served a function in maintaining the current family system was explored. It was evident that they prevented her from leaving her mother, whom she saw as needing to be looked after. Mother feared that Jane would follow Rachel and go and live with father. It emerged that before Rachel left home she had behaved in a seriously delinquent manner, so that moving to be with father was virtually forced on mother by her inability to control her. Jane's symptoms also served to keep father involved with his family in mutual concern with his ex-wife. It sometimes seemed as if Jane wanted the family to be reconstituted so that she could leave home without her mother being left entirely on her own. In the four sessions, when Mr Morgan or Rachel were also present, it was very obvious that both undermined Mrs Morgan's confidence and authority with Jane. Mrs Morgan was made to look incompetent.

During this period Jane lost weight rapidly and it dropped to 35kg. The psychiatrist's attempts to put mother in charge of Jane failed, as did interventions aimed at increasing Jane's independence from her mother. It seemed likely that Jane would need readmission soon.

## Reassessment

Jane's anorexia has been managed within the context of her family and the information made available by this approach has modified aspects of the original aetiological hypothesis. However, she has deteriorated in spite of the psychiatrist using this information. The reader is invited to reformulate Jane's problem in order to develop a more useful management strategy.

*Diagnosis*

This remains anorexia nervosa.

*Aetiology*

It is essential to establish what factors have perpetuated Jane's symptoms. It seems clear that family factors have been important in this, partly because of the additional information gathered and partly from the fact that Jane deteriorated markedly when her father and sister undermined her mother's responsibility for her.

It has become clear that both parents have had considerable difficulty in separating from their children. Jane's father has travelled over regularly from the USA to see them and on this occasion he has given up all of his holiday in order to do this. Not only has Rachel gone to the USA to live with her father, but it also seems she needed to be 'delinquent' in order to escape from her mother. Jane's mother now fears that Jane will also abandon her for her father and this has been reinforced to some extent by the way in which Rachel and her father have undermined her in the family sessions.

If Jane were to go to the USA with her father, her mother would then feel she had lost both of her daughters. This concern for her mother might have been sufficient to cause Jane's relapse, particularly if coupled with an equal wish to be with her father.

However, Jane did not appear to be trying to get away from her mother; in fact, the effect of her illness has been to reconstitute the family. Although this might be seen as an understandable hope in the child of a divorced couple, it is unusual for such a hope to be maintained for 15 years, unless at least one of the parents has failed to accept the divorce 'emotionally'.

There is some evidence that Mrs Morgan is the one who may have failed to come to terms with the divorce. Jane has said that she felt her mother still missed her father and Mrs Morgan expressed resentment about her ex-husband's impending return to the USA. On the other hand, Mr Morgan appears less likely to fill this role and seems to have suffered more from the loss of his children. He has certainly been consistent in his efforts to maintain contact with them.

It is possible that Jane remaining at home has maintained her mother's relationship with her ex-husband and that her illness and subsequent dependence on her mother has reinforced this.

## Management

It follows from this line of thinking that Jane's mother should be faced with her failure to 'emotionally' divorce her ex-husband and be encouraged to come to terms with this. This might involve her re-establishing a direct relationship with him that would exclude Jane.

Mrs Morgan will also need support and encouragement to withstand her ex-husband's undermining manoeuvres, if she is to deal with her fear that Jane will leave her for him.

Finally, if Jane continues to lose weight in spite of these interventions, she will need to be readmitted to hospital and a new management strategy developed.

## Further information

Jane's weight will continue to need monitoring.

The psychiatrist will need to observe closely the effect on Jane and her family of any interventions. Their response will determine whether to pursue the management outlined above, whether and how it should be modified, or whether it should be abandoned.

## Prognosis

If this formulation is correct then Jane should begin to improve. However, because of the hypothesized family dynamic, any improvement is likely to be met by a resistance within the family. In this case it might be expected that her father would make stronger efforts to undermine his ex-wife.

## Postscript

The psychiatrist undertook the management outlined above and spent a considerable period of time exploring and underlining Mrs Morgan's strengths.

The loss of her husband was discussed at some length and means were explored for her to negotiate a direct relationship with him that did not involve Jane. Mrs Morgan began to exercise more control over Jane's eating. However, as she began to gain weight Mr Morgan made an open attempt to separate her from her mother. He said the treatment was ineffective and he had therefore made arrangements for Jane to be seen by a famous specialist in the USA. Mrs Morgan had by now sufficient authority to resist her ex-husband's plans and Jane decided that she could not live with a father who was 'so domineering'.

Over the next four months Jane continued to gain weight and nine months after leaving hospital she had reached 45kg. She found a new job that she enjoyed and began to go out with a boyfriend, and was now able to discuss her uncertainties about the latter with her mother. A friend offered to share a flat with her but Jane was uncertain what to do about this. Although her mother said it was 'probably a good idea', her tone of voice showed that she was clearly unhappy about the possibility. Jane decided not to move out at this time.

# Chapter 6

# *A Domestic Dispute*

## *Mr Rogers*

The police telephoned to request assessment of Mr Rogers who was arrested following a domestic dispute. He was seen at the police station.

### Presenting complaint

The previous week, when both Mr Rogers and his partner were at home, he had cooked the evening meal and started drinking early in the evening. He thought he then drank between six and eight cans of normal-strength lager in total. He recalled having an argument over a television programme, because he was annoyed at being criticized for his choice of programme, but was unable to remember the details of what was said. He remembered going to bed in the early hours of the morning. After going to the bathroom he pushed his partner, Mr Amaro, away from him, because 'he wouldn't let go of the argument'. He thought he may have caught him in the face with his nail. He next remembered falling asleep and then being woken by his friend, Harry, who had come to visit at his partner's behest. When he became aware that his partner had telephoned the police he left the house with Harry, because 'I wanted to avoid any trouble'. 'Once I had sorted my head out', around lunchtime, he went to the police station and gave himself up. He was arrested and detained pending a psychiatric review, as he seemed 'a little odd', and the police were concerned that he might again be violent towards his partner.

Mr Rogers felt there was nothing really wrong with him except from feeling 'a bit edgy', and 'perhaps drinking a little too much alcohol from time to time'. He said that he and Mr Amaro had a good relationship, and although they argued occasionally, there had never been any violence before.

Mr Rogers also volunteered that he was the victim of an assault two years previously; he and Mr Amaro were at home when he was assaulted and robbed. He had CS gas sprayed in his face, was handcuffed and punched repeatedly. His nose and teeth were broken, and they were both threatened with being shot. The perpetrators stole £10,000 in cash and had not been found. Shortly afterwards, he moved house to escape the frightening memories, bought a guard dog, and arranged for a closed-circuit television surveillance system to be fitted outside his house. He felt that this experience had probably made him more wary of people.

## Family history

Mr Rogers' father had died 20 years before, aged 59. He worked as a civil engineer and was described as 'very strict, excessively so, but never violent or threatening'. His 74-year-old mother was a cook, remained fit and was living in Scotland. He had two sisters and one brother, and all his siblings were married and had children. He maintained contact with his older brother, a doctor, and his youngest sister, who worked in catering. His mother recently told him that she suffered a nervous breakdown when she was in her 20s, just before he was born. There was no other family history of mental illness.

## Personal history

Mr Rogers was born in Edinburgh. He described normal developmental milestones and attended school until the age of 16. He enjoyed his junior school and was a good pupil at his comprehensive school. He played football and rugby for the school, never truanted, and was well behaved with no disciplinary problems. He left school without taking any examinations, as he was keen to get away from home. He then joined the army, but found his basic training arduous, both physically and mentally. He described a tour of duty in Northern Ireland to Crossmaglen in the 1980s where he saw many people shot and killed, including friends. He left the army after finishing this tour, when he was 26.

He married when he was 19 and divorced three years later. Initially he said this was because his partner found it difficult while he was away on army exercises. Later in the interview he attributed it to the fact that he realized he was homosexual after a gay experience during his off-duty time. He had no children and was not in contact with his ex-partner. He also said he did not keep in touch with any of his friends from his army days.

Afterwards, Mr Rogers worked in the building trade for a year and subsequently applied to join the 'Sabre Watch' security services. He worked for them as a night security guard in a large retail depot and enjoyed this. However, during his second year there he was exposed to an extremely unpleasant and frightening experience, which resulted in his leaving. The fire alarm in the toy warehouse went off one night while he was on duty. When he arrived there he saw some smoke and opened the side door with the emergency key to assess the extent of the fire. He saw dense smoke and felt intense heat coming from the building, but could not locate any obvious source of the fire. He could also hear someone shouting from inside the building, and decided to go into the building to find the person who was shouting. The situation was far worse than he had imagined and he had to start crawling on his hands and knees. He then came across two men; one had a towel covering his face, and the other was not moving and appeared to be dead. He struggled to move both of them out of the building, but they were too heavy. Eventually he struggled out with the man with the towel. By the time he managed to find his way out the fire brigade had arrived. A fire crew with breathing apparatus retrieved the body inside the building and the two men were given resuscitation. However, they were both dead. Sometime later there was a formal investigation, and he was commended for his bravery.

Following this episode he experienced a gradual decline in his well-being. He found it difficult to sleep and started drinking alcohol with increasing frequency. One month later he had an argument with his supervisor, left his job, and moved to another security firm. To begin with he did not feel there was any problem, but within a year he found that things had 'come to a head'. He saw his general practitioner at the beginning of the year, and was told that he was suffering from depression. He was then referred to the practice counsellor, and a month later he went on sick leave. Subsequently he started a small business helping a friend sell videos, but found it difficult to cope and stopped after a few months. Since then he had not been able to work.

Mr Rogers had been living with his current partner, Mr Amaro, for the last three years. He described him as 'highly strung' and said that they often argued, but never fought.

At the time of his arrest he had built up significant debts and there was a possible repossession order on his house. He had no income apart from his incapacity benefit. Mr Amaro did not work.

## Past medical history

Nothing significant was mentioned.

## Past psychiatric history

Mr Rogers was not taking any medication at the present time. However, 18 months previously he was prescribed an antidepressant, fluoxetine, 20–40mgs per day, and he continued this until about three months before. He did not think it had helped him in any way.

## Alcohol and drugs

He said that since his days in the army he had always been part of a drinking culture, he always drank with other people and had never tried to give it up. He said he had never used any illicit drugs. While working for the security firm he kept himself fit by exercising regularly.

## Criminal history

Mr Rogers' first contact with the police was two years previously. 'I clipped my partner around his head' after an argument, and Mr Amaro called the police. He received a conditional discharge of 12 months.

## Previous personality

Mr Rogers said he had considered himself a cheerful and outgoing man who enjoyed the company of his friends and a good drink. He liked reading the paper, usually *The Sun*, every day. He had also enjoyed his work and was often commended on his 'smart appearance and disciplined approach'. All these areas had suffered since he stopped work.

## Mental state examination

### Appearance and general behaviour

Mr Rogers was a white, slim, clean-shaven man with tattooed forearms who exhibited a fine tremor in his hands at rest. He established a good rapport and made direct eye contact. As the interview progressed he became increasingly settled, but became fidgety and tearful when he talked about the fire and the associated traumatic incidents.

### Speech

Mr Rogers gave a fluent and coherent account of himself, his background, and the circumstances leading up to his arrest.

### Mood

Mr Rogers felt very miserable. He described disturbed sleep, poor concentration, low sexual interest and loss of appetite; over the last two years he had lost two stones in weight. He experienced a pervasive feeling of sadness for himself and his partner. Sometimes he found himself crying for no obvious reason, although this could be set off by images on the television or photographs around the house. On occasions he had thoughts about killing himself by hanging or taking tablets. However, he had not acted on these because 'I can't bear the thought of leaving my partner and my dogs behind'.

Mr Rogers also described increased irritability with more frequent loss of temper than ever in the past. He accepted that this might be due to his excessive alcohol consumption, and said he recognized that drinking was a problem rather than a solution to his difficulties. He said he had no intention to harm his partner, and was ashamed of being in his current predicament.

### Thought content

Throughout the interview Mr Rogers mentioned how uncomfortable he felt in company and that he went out of his way to avoid crowded places. He also avoided any enclosed spaces. He always felt anxious, even at home, and described this as 'feeling very jumpy'. Whenever he did go out he found himself scanning the faces of everyone walking towards him, looking for the people responsible for the burglary.

### Abnormal beliefs and interpretations of events

Mr Rogers avoided going into the road where he lived when he was assaulted. He had a constant feeling that 'something dangerous is going to happen to me or my family' and constantly needed to be 'on the lookout'.

### Abnormal experiences

He described experiencing 'flashbacks' to the fire and the assault two or three times a week. During these episodes, which lasted up to half an hour, he saw himself lying on the floor at home, choking with smoke or being assaulted on the floor.

### Cognitive state

Brief cognitive testing revealed no significant abnormalities of his attention or of his short- or long-term memory.

### Self-appraisal

Mr Rogers said he was told that his nerves were affected by his frightening experiences. He knew this was called a post-traumatic stress disorder.

Mr Rogers scored 48 on the 'Beck Depression Inventory' (30 or above is indicative of a severe depressive illness) and 60 on the revised 'Impact of Events Scale' related to his experiences of the assault and burglary (an average score of sufferers of post-traumatic stress disorder is 39.5).

## Physical examination

This was not performed at the police station.

A collateral history was not available; Mr Amaro was not at home and his mobile phone was set to the answer phone. The police were able to confirm that his partner had alleged assault and there was evidence of some facial bruising. They also added that Mr Rogers had a previous record of assault on his partner.

## Preliminary assessment

Until the fire, Mr Rogers' life and career were reasonably uneventful. When he was in the army he had coped with the considerable pressures of being in Northern Ireland. He completed his commission successfully and left with good references. This was maintained when he worked as a security guard, where he again established a reputation as a reliable and presentable employee. His difficulties began following the fire, which was distressing and life threatening. He slowly deteriorated and eventually left security work. A further life-threatening life episode two years later seems to have been critical in re-awakening his symptoms and setting off a precipitous decline in his mental health. The attack on his partner occurred when Mr Rogers had been drinking heavily, and he was unable to recall all the details of this event.

### Diagnosis

Mr Rogers is suffering from post-traumatic stress disorder (PTSD). This is a unique diagnosis, since being exposed to a profound and unusual traumatic event is the essential component that distinguishes it from depression and anxiety. In this example there were two such events, the warehouse fire and the robbery. Both of these were characteristic of this disorder, in that they seriously threatened his life and he was helpless; it is likely that the first event precipitated the onset, which was further aggravated by the second event. His symptoms also bear directly on these events. He has recurrent and intrusive recollections of the fire, reminders of this event evoke marked distress, and memories colour his nightmares. Since the robbery he has been in a constant hyper-vigilant state, constantly scanning faces and attempting to avoid contact with people. In addition, he avoids returning to where it took place. He also has symptoms of increased arousal, insomnia, irritability, and difficulty in concentrating. This post-trauma irritability could account for the assaults on his partner, all of which post-date the warehouse fire. His social and occupational function has become seriously impaired by these changes, and has been present for at least four years. His illness therefore falls at the severe end of the spectrum.

Mr Rogers also suffers from depression. This is characterized by his low mood, loss of sleep, diminished appetite, poor concentration, suicidal ideation and his hopelessness about his future. These symptoms are too severe and long-standing to be explained by the PTSD and have resulted in his withdrawal from the social activities that he previously enjoyed.

Mr Rogers was also using alcohol to try and ameliorate some of the above symptoms and he fulfils the criteria for alcohol abuse, although falling short of a full alcohol dependent syndrome.

*Aetiology*

Mr Rogers may have a genetic predisposition to develop a depressive illness or a stress reaction, as his mother had a 'breakdown' in the past. Although he described a happy atmosphere at home, he also said discipline was strict and he was keen to leave home and join the army 'as soon as possible'. This might make one wonder about the quality of his relationship with his father. However, he fitted in well with the army's structured life and tolerated aversive experiences in Northern Ireland without any notable disturbance. This suggests that he was able to cope with considerable levels of stress. It may be that the support of his friends within the army helped diffuse the experience. His present difficulties stem from his stress reaction secondary to the fire whilst he was working as a security guard. He described clear symptoms of PTSD after this episode, and it is likely that these were fuelled by his sense of guilt at leaving one of the men behind in the smoke. The robbery and assault sound sufficiently frightening to have triggered an emotional reaction on their own account. In the context of his experience of the fire they are therefore particularly likely to have exacerbated the original symptoms and precipitated his current depression, which may have relapsed since the discontinuation of antidepressant therapy over the last few months.

He said he was gay, and did not make any further references to his sexuality. There is often little tolerance in 'macho' institutions such as the army and one could speculate as to whether this was the reason why he left. Certainly, he said he did not keep in touch with any army friends.

The current difficulties are maintained by alcohol abuse and this is also a major contribution to the friction in his relationship, which has culminated in his arrest. He has always drunk alcohol to excess and much of his social life revolves around 'the pub'. This is an expected part of army life and also associated with the type of employment he then followed. He was therefore particularly at risk of increasing his alcohol intake when faced with additional stress.

*Further information*

Ideally, a collateral history from his partner is required, both to corroborate the respective account of the assault and to have an independent view of his difficulties.

The police have requested a report focusing on the likelihood of any further violence and it will therefore need to incorporate a risk assessment. A detailed history from informants as well as Mr Rogers is therefore required. It should pay special attention to substance abuse and an account of any previous criminal activities, and include an assessment of his intelligence, personality and sexual feelings (where appropriate). His mental state needs to be assessed over several interviews to clarify the relationship between any offences, or threats of such, and his mental state at the time, his attitude towards treatment and his previous response to therapy. Finally, there should be a detailed description of the present offence, focusing on any predisposing and precipitating factors that may be revealed, and his emotional and cognitive state at the time it occurred.

In Mr Rogers' case, we have some of this information, but lack other important data. In particular we have only a sketchy picture of the alleged assault, because he said he was unable to remember any details. This may well be true because he has been frank in his descriptions of other events in his personal history, and acknowledges his alcohol consumption. The severity of the alleged assault also seems to bear his story out, since the police report only noted superficial bruising to his partner's face.

*Management*

In the short term, the police want to know if he is safe to release on bail. Longer-term issues are the appropriate treatment of his PTSD, depression and alcohol abuse.

Overall management will require regular outpatient contact to provide support, to consider and recommence appropriate antidepressant treatment and to assess his suitability for specialized treatment for his traumatic stress disorder. In addition it would allow the psychiatrist to focus on reducing his alcohol consumption, either in the clinic or by referral to a specialized drugs and alcohol team. If a sound therapeutic relationship develops, the relevance of his sexuality to his predicament might also be explored in more depth.

On the basis of the information so far obtained, it would be difficult to suggest that his illness was of sufficient severity, or his dangerousness to his partner was such, that he should continue to be detained in hospital or the police station. One option would be to allow him to be released on bail, with advice to stay away from his partner.

*Prognosis*

This depends to a considerable extent upon the accuracy of the information obtained so far. However, it does sound as if Mr Rogers is suffering from psychiatric disorders which are treatable, and that he will be safe to leave the police station, provided certain safeguards are met.

## Further details

Mr Amaro eventually responded to his mobile phone, and said he was willing to come to the police station. It was decided to delay implementing the management plan until further information was acquired. Contact was also made with Mr Rogers' general practitioner, who was able to fax a brief history of his contact with him.

### Interview with Mr Amaro

Mr Amaro confirmed that he had been arguing with Mr Rogers about the television. He had been more irritable than usual, and thought this was due to the pressure he was under at the time, because their house was due to be repossessed on the Wednesday of that week. He felt he had to sit with Mr Rogers until 4 a.m., because he seemed so angry and didn't wish him to go to bed. When they did go to bed Mr Rogers went to the bathroom, returned to the bedroom and 'slapped me, out of the blue'. He then went to sleep. He went on to say that he was 'clearly out of it' and 'didn't know what he was doing'. In the morning he phoned Harry, a friend of the couple, told him that Mr Rogers had 'flipped during the night' and said it would be a good idea to check up on him while Mr Amaro went to stay with friends. Later in the morning, in response to Mr Rogers' telephone calls, he returned home and 'as I came through the door he grabbed my jacket and threw it on the floor' in a very aggressive fashion. He again left to go to a friend's house, from where he called the police. Later, he returned home and was subsequently placed in a refuge for two nights.

Before this episode they had frequent arguments on a weekly basis, but during the last two years there had never been any physical altercation. Mr Rogers drank alcohol regularly. Mr Amaro made it clear how worried they both were about the repossession of the house that they shared.

By the time he was interviewed Mr Amaro decided that he didn't wish to pursue the assault charge and withdrew his allegations. He said he was happy to return home with Mr Rogers, provided he take up the offer of help and reduce his drinking.

### General practice records

The records revealed that Mr Rogers had initially been prescribed Prozac (fluoxetine), which he had found helpful with his depression while he was taking it. He has later prescribed sertraline, but stopped this after one week, following adverse side effects. He was then given amitriptyline, 20mgs per day, for a very brief period.

There was also a letter from the counsellor who had been seeing Mr Rogers:

> Mr Rogers told me that he did not suffer any untoward physical or mental sequelae as a result of his time in Northern Ireland. He reported significant difficulties after the fire incident, following which he developed insomnia, flashbacks, tearfulness and irritability. He told me that he was debriefed following the incident, but did not take up the offer of any formal counselling because he did not perceive any problems. He described a gradual decline since then. He assaulted a colleague in the following year and had to change employment. He described himself as 'slipping down' and was unable to travel on the underground any more because of claustrophobia. He decided not to go driving on his own because he was unable to concentrate fully. He told me that the thing that finally precipitated his leaving work was the death of his grandfather, then he was placed on long-term sick leave. He has a very vivid memory of spending three months during that time sitting in his garden drinking alcohol and imagining 'ways of ending it all'. He sought help at this stage and was treated with antidepressants and had contact with Alcoholics Anonymous. The burglary occurred in the context of this anxiety and, he believes, made his mental condition much worse.
>
> Mr Rogers described his continued heavy alcohol usage, of between 130 and 140 units of alcohol a week. He exclusively drank beer and he drank on his own, sometimes following a binge pattern where he may start drinking in the morning and continue for two or three days. He told me that he rarely goes out drinking socially, any more. He reports only one day of abstinence since stopping work.
>
> My view is that he is suffering from a post-traumatic stress disorder and he is willing to work with me on addressing this.

## Reassessment

### Diagnosis

The additional information confirms the diagnosis of PTSD and depression with suicidal ideation and somatic features. It also highlights the significance of his use of alcohol, which changed from the previous social pattern and became increasingly isolated and harmful, verging on dependence. The depressive episode developed after the PTSD, and could be considered secondary to, or part of, it.

## Aetiology

The main aetiological factors outlined previously have been substantiated. However, the significance of his grandfather's death has now come to light.

## Management

The initial management plan should now be followed. A sedative antidepressant should be prescribed and an outpatient appointment arranged. He should also be given a contact telephone number for the local community mental health team and a home assessment should be undertaken if he fails to keep his appointment. He will require a physical examination and appropriate investigations, and his alcohol consumption needs to be monitored. He should also be advised to re-establish contact with Alcoholics Anonymous, and the possibility of referral to the local drug and alcohol team should be considered if there is no improvement. In the longer term, provided he cooperates with treatment, he can be assessed for cognitive behavioural therapy by the psychology service.

## Prognosis

Mr Rogers is likely to make a full recovery, given his previous personality, the stability of his relationship with his partner and the fact that his recent deterioration was contingent upon a series of major life events.

## Postscript

Mr Rogers was released from the police station and the assault charge was dropped. He accepted the offer to be seen in outpatients in a week's time. Six months later Mr Rogers had improved considerably, and Mr Amaro confirmed this. In particular, his mood had lifted; he was also much calmer, no longer irritable and sleeping well.

These reported changes were apparent in his mental state, which was essentially normal. He said he had easily managed to reduce his alcohol intake to recommended limits within three weeks of release. No further conflicts were reported. The local psychology service offered him a place for treatment, but by then he felt completely recovered and discontinued contact with the community mental health team.

Chapter 7

# A Blackout at Work

## Mr Pillay

**Presenting complaint**

Mr Pillay, a 46-year-old Mauritian of Indian extraction, was referred to the Department of Psychological Medicine in a General Hospital following his admission to a general ward. He had been admitted from the Accident and Emergency Department following a 'black-out' in a photographic laboratory where he worked. He was found deeply unconscious by a workmate but had sustained no injury.

The referring physician gave the following account of the admission.

On arrival at the hospital Mr Pillay was found to be pyrexial, shivering, agitated, tremulous and disorientated and was diagnosed as suffering from a chest infection and an acute confusional state. On admission to the ward he showed clouding of consciousness, difficulty in attending to questions and an inability to register what was going on about him. He was grossly disorientated in time and place. A physical examination revealed he had a temperature of 39°C and there was evidence of consolidation of the lungs. A chest X-ray revealed a picture of bronchopneumonia.

Mr Pillay remained confused for the next three days. He was found to wander around the ward looking for 'the singers' and complained that people were getting at him. One nurse was accused of administering poisons to him. Treatment with ampicillin for the chest infection was accompanied by a resolution of the fever and in addition he was sedated with chlordiazepoxide for five days.

On the fourth day he was able to give a history. At this stage he admitted to drinking 'two pints of beer and one eighth of a bottle of whisky' per day. Liver function tests showed a raised gamma GT level (45IU/L). Mr Pillay was seen on the medical ward by a social worker. He complained to her of problems at work but said that otherwise he had no difficulties in his life. He said that he had many friends, 'too many', and that drinking would not be a problem in the future. An appointment was offered for the psychiatric outpatient department two weeks later and Mr Pillay accepted it to reassure everyone that everything was all right.

Mr Pillay was subsequently discharged from his inpatient stay, and when he arrived for his outpatient appointment the following history was obtained.

He had few complaints. Those that he had were exclusively concerned with his work as a technician in a dark room. The air conditioner had recently broken down and after sharing a confined space with two co-workers for a day he felt 'jittery' and as if his head was 'exploding'.

When asked directly, Mr Pillay said that he had been drinking regularly from the age of 19 but that his intake had increased over the past six years since he had started his current job. The amount of alcohol which he admitted consuming was as stated during his stay on the ward. On occasions, though, he said he might have drunk a quarter of a bottle of spirits. Mr Pillay admitted to a morning drink 'rarely' and also to some morning tremulousness and dry retching 'occasionally', although more frequently over the past few months. He denied any 'black-outs' in the past or any lapses of memory. Mr Pillay said he normally drank every day but when he developed a cough and fever with his chest infection he stopped. This was a few days before his admission to hospital. Since discharge from the hospital ten days earlier he said he had drunk three beers but no spirits.

## Family history

Mr Pillay's father was aged 76 and a plantation manager in Mauritius. Although fit, Mr Pillay described him as a 'very heavy drinker'. His mother was aged 68 and well.

He had two brothers and one sister. Both his brothers were in Mauritius and one was older than the patient. They were both successful in their careers, one a civil servant and the other an accountant. His sister, aged 34, was the youngest child; she lived with her husband and two children in London, a few miles from Mr Pillay's home.

His family was 'close' and relationships had always been harmonious. He spoke of his parents in idealistic terms, and said he was brought up with much 'love, care and affection'. They corresponded regularly, but Mr Pillay had not visited Mauritius since his arrival in England six years previously. He saw his sister most weekends, until three months previously when she had her second child.

There was no family history of mental disorder and his father had never required medical attention on account of his drinking. An uncle was mentioned, now dead from a cause unknown to the patient, who was also a heavy drinker.

## Personal history

There had been some complications surrounding Mr Pillay's birth. He did not know their exact nature but he remembered being told that little hope had been held for his survival. Apart from this, his childhood had been unremarkable. He had a tendency to keep to himself. His family had regarded him as 'independent' from an early age and had commented on a 'stubborn streak' in his make-up.

Mr Pillay went to a highly regarded private school in Mauritius and matriculated at the age of 19. He was a serious and ambitious student who was expected to do well in the future.

On leaving school Mr Pillay went to work in the civil service. After five years he became private secretary to a government minister, a post which he held for four years. He then moved to a merchant bank where he held an administrative position of some responsibility for ten years. Then, at the age of 39, Mr Pillay left the bank, for reasons which he explained vaguely, one of them being a change of location.

At this time he decided to come to England where his sister was already living. He said that he had always had a special interest in, and flair for, design, and for the first year after his arrival he worked as an interior decorator, but with only modest success. Mr Pillay obtained his present job as a laboratory technician in a specialist photographic firm six years previously, through the agency of a friend. The laboratory dealt with quality photographic reproductions and Mr Pillay worked mainly in a highly organized darkroom. For the past year or so he had become less enthusiastic about his work and often complained about the cramped and stuffy conditions. He suggested a number of possible improvements, but to no avail. He thought his employers were 'very satisfied' with his work and that his job had never been threatened. Mr Pillay had never married because the idea of marriage had never appealed to him. He had, however, had a number of short-lived affairs, which he termed 'illicit', as some had been with married women. He did not have a current partner.

He lived in a rented flat that he had decorated himself and of which he was proud. He said that he was a 'gregarious' man who had 'lots of friends'. The impression was given that they drank together, although he was at pains to point out that none were excessive drinkers.

## Past medical history

Mr Pillay had malaria when he was 7 and viral pneumonia at the age of 26. He also had an episode of 'rheumatic pains' in the legs a year previously, for which he did not seek treatment.

## Past psychiatric history

None was elicited.

## Previous personality

Mr Pillay described himself as a 'slightly nervous' man who generally felt in control of his life. He denied ever feeling low spirited. He said that he tended to become 'impatient if things are not done right'. This somewhat perfectionist trait had led him to complain about the organization of the laboratory at work. Mr Pillay spent much time in meticulously decorating his flat. He described decoration and carpentry as his main interests and he was frequently employed by acquaintances to do odd jobs of this kind. He indicated that he expected a high standard of moral behaviour from other people and that he tried to maintain similar high standards for himself. However, he found it difficult to assert himself and tended to back down in arguments. He used to read novels but had not done so for a year or so. Although brought up as a Christian he was a non-believer, as he could find no 'convincing evidence' to support such beliefs.

Mr Pillay had never been in trouble with the police. He smoked 30–40 cigarettes a day and he denied taking any illicit drugs.

## Physical examination

On his discharge from hospital there were no abnormal physical findings. This was not performed again.

## Mental state examination
### *Appearance and general behaviour*

Mr Pillay was a small, thin man with his hair immaculately combed in such a way as to conceal an advanced state of baldness. He was well spoken and pleasant at all times and displayed a very deferential manner to the psychiatrist, frequently addressing him as 'sir'.

During the interview he was politely evasive and gave the impression that he was painting a brighter picture than the real one. Most questions touching on potentially sensitive areas (such as leaving Mauritius or sexual feelings) were answered briefly or side-tracked into less emotionally charged ones. This was done in an ostensibly respectful manner but his obvious discomfort and reluctance made the interviewer feel that further probing at this stage would not prove rewarding. There was a powerful sense that only issues lying close to the surface were to be discussed.

Mr Pillay looked uncomfortable and was almost constantly fidgety.

### *Speech*
This was fluent and spontaneous.

*Mood*

Mr Pillay denied any depressive feelings and said he was optimistic about the future. He expressed no feelings of self-reproach. He admitted to feeling tense at times but made light of this. Somatic accompaniments to his anxiety were denied.

*Thought content*

This was mainly concerned with difficulties at work, which he believed could now be remedied. He repeatedly referred to 'the facts' and said he was pleased that his employer was finally taking some notice of his complaints.

*Abnormal beliefs and interpretations of events*

There were none currently, but Mr Pillay vaguely recalled harbouring the belief that he was the subject of persecution during his hospital admission.

*Cognitive state*

Cognitive testing revealed no abnormality of memory or intellectual functioning. Digit span up to seven numbers forwards and five numbers backwards was executed without difficulty. A name and address were perfectly recalled after five minutes and Mr Pillay was very well informed about current news events.

*Self-appraisal*

Mr Pillay conceded that he might have been drinking too much before but he was now confident that it would never be a problem again. He believed that the symptoms necessitating his admission to hospital were entirely the result of his chest infection and claimed that no one had ever told him that they might be related to alcohol. The suggestion that these were recognized symptoms of alcohol addiction and withdrawal seemed to surprise him. Armed with this new knowledge, he said, he would be even more determined to control his drinking.

When it was advised that abstinence was the wisest course on which to embark, Mr Pillay said that he could not accept the idea of stopping alcohol completely. At times he gave indications that he was unsure about whether he needed help. The idea was never totally dismissed but when he was asked to specify what he might need help with, he talked mainly about 'problems in the dark room'. When asked whether he was content with the way he was managing other aspects of his life he answered affirmatively.

At the end of the interview Mr Pillay was asked whether he minded if the doctor spoke to his sister in order to learn more about his situation. He replied that he did not wish to 'burden' her with his problem, especially as she had recently had a baby. After further discussion he persistently but politely forbade any contact. He also said that he did not want to impose on his friends and that he would be unhappy if his employer were to know any details of his troubles.

## Assessment

Mr Pillay is a 46-year-old man referred following admission to a medical ward because of a 'black-out' and the development of a seriously disturbed mental state. His symptoms resolved after a few days and he was referred to a psychiatrist for an assessment of his drinking behaviour.

Having clarified the importance of alcohol in his presentation, the fundamental difficulty confronting the psychiatrist is to communicate his understanding of the problems of alcohol dependence to Mr Pillay in such a way as to facilitate his maximum cooperation with treatment.

### Diagnosis

The clinical picture displayed by Mr Pillay on admission to the ward was typical of a withdrawal state with delirium and possible convulsions in someone with an alcohol dependence syndrome. For two to three days his consciousness was clouded, he was disorientated in time and place, he was unable to register events going on about him and there was also evidence of agitation, auditory hallucinations and fleeting persecutory delusions. In Mr Pillay's case there was an obvious physical disorder, namely bronchopneumonia. However, this is unlikely to cause such a florid confusional state as this, except in the very young and the aged.

It is likely in Mr Pillay's case that alcohol played an important role. Withdrawal from alcohol in a physically dependent person may result in an acute confusional state termed delirium tremens. His drinking has certainly been sustained for many years and the raised gamma GT level in his liver function tests supports this. He admitted to morning tremulousness 'occasionally', which is an early feature of physical dependence on alcohol. Dry retching in the morning also points to excessive alcohol consumption. Although the 'black-out' was not witnessed, he was found to be deeply unconscious and was confused afterwards, and convulsions often usher in the florid mental disturbances of delirium tremens. It is therefore likely that this was an epileptic fit. The history also suggests that Mr Pillay, as a consequence of his chest infection, had reduced his alcohol intake and was therefore experiencing a state of relative withdrawal from alcohol. The marked agitation and tremulousness observed are part of the picture of delirium tremens.

Mr Pillay is either underestimating his consumption of alcohol or he is dissimulating. His failure to recall that he had been told his symptoms were associated with alcohol points to an ability on his part to 'deny' unpleasant memories. The personal history he gave was superficial, and this makes the search for other evidence of a drinking problem, such as a history of psychological or social impairment, difficult. There are a few clues, but their interpretation involves a large degree of inference. Mr Pillay's life appears to have gone into decline, most obviously in his work history. After doing well at school he seemed to occupy responsible jobs in government and later, in a bank, which called for the exercise of administrative skills. He then left Mauritius for reasons that are obscure and he now finds himself in the relatively unskilled position of a dark room technician. He considered himself ambitious and hard working, and it may be that his departure from Mauritius was related to a drinking problem even then. This suspicion is strengthened by Mr Pillay's vague account of why he left. It is difficult to gauge from the history whether there has been deterioration in his personal relationships. Finally, the 'rheumatic pains' that he described as having occurred a year ago were possibly the calf tenderness that alcoholics commonly experience.

There is no evidence that Mr Pillay suffers from a psychiatric illness, such as depression, to which his drinking might be secondary.

To summarize, Mr Pillay has suffered from an episode of acute organic confusion in which alcohol withdrawal has played a major role with a contribution from a chest infection. There is evidence that he drinks excessively and that he is physically dependent on alcohol. There is lesser evidence of a social decline, which might have been a consequence of drinking. Apart from some evidence of liver damage on admission to hospital there were no other physical or neuropsychiatric complications.

*Aetiology*

Those factors causing the acute confusional state have already been discussed. The precise pathophysiology caused by excessive drinking and which results in delirium tremens is unknown. Most cases commence two to three days after abstinence from alcohol and may be preceded by one or a series of epileptic fits. There is a significant association between delirium tremens and physical disorders, such as pneumonia, each of which may exacerbate the other. Alcoholic tremulousness is also a symptom of alcohol withdrawal, which occurs after a short period of abstinence, even overnight. Morning nausea and vomiting are usually attributed to alcoholic gastritis but they may also be of central nervous system origin and related to withdrawal.

The fact that Mr Pillay has shown evidence of physical dependence on alcohol indicates that he drinks heavily and that this has been sustained for a long time. The history obtained is not a very satisfactory one in terms of the information it provides which might have a bearing on aetiological factors. Few facts have been adduced which are helpful in understanding why Mr Pillay drinks heavily and one is forced at this stage to make a number of inferences which receive only limited support.

Both Mr Pillay's father and an uncle were heavy drinkers, and a familial 'transmission' of heavy drinking is common. However, although there is some evidence of a genetic predisposition to the development of physical dependence on alcohol, this is difficult to disentangle from the psychological influences existing in a home where a parent is a heavy drinker.

Mr Pillay does not appear to have been drinking heavily as a consequence of a psychiatric disorder such as depression. One looks, therefore, for personality vulnerabilities or difficult life circumstances which might predispose him to seek gratification or relief of tension in alcohol. With someone who has a long drinking history it is often difficult to distinguish difficulties that lead to drinking from those which are a consequence of drinking. Comment has already been made on Mr Pillay's work record. It is possible that the decline noted was a consequence of excessive drinking but it is also possible that a failure to achieve the success he wished for, due perhaps to personal limitations, might have led him to drink more.

Mr Pillay described some personality traits that could be seen as potentially problematic. He said that he tended to be an anxious man and his tension was indeed obvious during the interview. The frustration he felt if things were 'not right' seems to be related to some perfectionist traits in his personality. This may well have contributed to some of his difficulties at work, where a mixture of impatience and unassertiveness appear to have inhibited him from acting more forcefully with regard to his complaints. His deferential manner, which seemed inappropriate to the psychiatrist and was such a striking feature during the interview, was consistent with his view of himself as someone who finds it difficult to be self-assertive. However, this contrasts with his resolute resistance to give permission for his sister to be contacted. Although it might be understandable in cultural terms, it could also reflect his stubbornness, which he has acknowledged.

Mr Pillay's social situation is problematical. He claimed to have many friends, yet he gave the impression of being isolated. It is difficult to specify where this impression derives from but a number of factors suggesting this have emerged. He described himself as a 'loner' in childhood. A specific friend was never mentioned during the interview, nor was there ever any reference to other people having any impact on his life. He gave the impression of being a very private person. This is consistent with his finding marriage undesirable and the absence of any long-term heterosexual relationships. The main supportive figure in his life seemed to have been his sister, with whom he spent most weekends. The fact that she had a baby recently might have a bearing on his having presented at this time, since it is conceivable that she had withdrawn some support from him as a result of this. She never made contact with a doctor to discuss her brother's condition and may not even have known about his illness. Finally, Mr Pillay appeared during the interview to be someone who could not relate comfortably to the doctor. Although allowance needs to be made for the threatening nature of an interview with a psychiatrist, as well as cultural style, Mr Pillay's difficulties seemed to be more profound. His defensiveness, although polite, made it difficult to warm to him. He gave the impression of detached aloofness and of inexperience in talking about himself with others. There was a striking absence of an easy social competence.

Many of the factors discussed above which might have a bearing on Mr Pillay's drinking are speculative in view of the meagre information available. However, some of the ideas raised will guide the psychiatrist in the type of information to seek when the next opportunity presents itself.

### Further information

There is clearly a need for more personal details. The exact extent to which alcohol has salience in Mr Pillay's life is unclear. Also the course of his life history and the effect that drinking has had on his work and social relationships need further exploration. Evidence is also necessary to evaluate the postulated role of personality factors in predisposing him to drink excessively. An informant, particularly his sister, would be the most helpful source of information, but at present this is barred by Mr Pillay. One will have to rely therefore on what can be learnt from further interviews with the patient himself.

A repeat of the liver function tests should be performed to check whether the gamma GT level has returned to normal.

More detailed psychological testing for cognitive impairment should be considered, as should an MRI scan. These would provide measures against which future testing might reveal deterioration. Any impairment demonstrated should be discussed with Mr Pillay since it might increase his motivation for treatment.

## Management

The major difficulty is Mr Pillay's apparent lack of motivation to seek help. The details of any treatment can only be worked out if he makes a commitment to give up drinking and this aim would be much more realistic if he could establish a therapeutic alliance with the doctor.

The absence of information about the extent to which drinking has interfered with Mr Pillay's life makes it difficult to decide on how much pressure should be exerted on him to accept treatment. He denies a significant impact on his level of functioning, although there is good evidence that he is physically dependent on alcohol. Because of this, one would want to encourage him to make a more realistic appraisal of his difficulties. Mr Pillay's failure to disclose important details is an important limitation in this task. There is a temptation to challenge him by saying that he is not very concerned to cooperate, to discharge him, and to suggest that he will be back soon enough.

However, another attempt might be made to enlist his cooperation. For this to have any hope of success, special attention will need to be paid to the relationship made with him and this will need to take account of some of the observations already discussed. The interviewer will have to be on guard against reacting to Mr Pillay's contradictory, submissive stubbornness with impatience, and will need to respect his privacy. The best approach might involve an implicit indication that the interview is not 'psychological' but 'factual'. Fewer 'Why did that happen?' and more 'What happened then?' questions would help to create a 'fact finding' atmosphere. The aim would be to construct a picture of an average day in Mr Pillay's life: what he does and with whom, when he drinks and what. 'Feelings' should be left out. At the end of the session a joint appraisal can be made of the 'facts of the case' and Mr Pillay invited to draw logical conclusions. Since he mentioned 'facts' a number of times during his first interview this approach might fit in better with his way of viewing the world. It is also important to inform him of the physical, psychological and social risks he faces with continued drinking.

If Mr Pillay were to agree to treatment it is difficult at this stage to suggest which type of treatment would prove most helpful to him. The treatment needs to be tailored to his particular needs and these are not clear. The goal should be abstinence in view of his physical dependence on alcohol. Long-term supportive measures will be necessary to help him achieve this and their nature would also depend on a fuller assessment of his specific difficulties. For example, he might need some help towards greater assertiveness in dealing with others. Medication, such as Antabuse, or support, as provided by Alcoholics Anonymous, might also play a role. However, given his social unease the latter might not prove acceptable to him.

If Mr Pillay elects not to accept the offer of treatment then it would be reasonable to leave him with the invitation to refer himself back if he should change his mind in the future.

*Prognosis*

It is always difficult to predict the outcome of alcohol dependency, however strong someone's motivation might appear. Even if treatment is eventually successful, it is frequently interrupted by relapses. A long-term view therefore needs to be taken, which allows a relationship with the therapist to develop regardless of any such vicissitudes. A confident prognosis cannot therefore be given in Mr Pillay's case. Unless he can change his attitude to his drinking it is likely that it will continue and that further complications such as withdrawal symptoms and liver damage will occur. Quite apart from his own lack of incentive to abstain is the apparent absence of people in his life who might encourage him to stop drinking. Mr Pillay has apparently shown some ability to control his drinking in the past since he has been able to sustain his job without interruption. However, if he continues in the same vein, it is very likely that more problems will arise.

This admission to hospital, however, may represent the first occasion on which Mr Pillay has had to confront his drinking. There is a small chance that it may result in a significant change in his behaviour without anyone else's help.

## Further details

Mr Pillay was given an appointment to return to the clinic one month later. The Christmas period intervened between the first and second visits.

When he was next seen in the clinic he said that he was very well except that he was 'virtually compelled' by his friends to have a 'brandy or two' over Christmas. He admitted also to a pint of Guinness on another occasion but was adamant that he had consumed no more. He remarked that he felt much better, that his appetite had improved and that he was now eating breakfast after getting up with a 'clear mind'. His work situation had also improved and a new rota had been established. His colleagues had been supportive and urged him to go out for a walk when 'the cell becomes too stuffy'. He had avoided his firm's Christmas parties and said, 'If I put my mind to it I could live without alcohol.' In the evenings he had visited his sister or his friends. They knew about his problems now and avoided drinking in his presence.

The pathology report indicated that his liver function tests had reverted to normal.

Mr Pillay said he did not need any further help, but agreed to come again in three months' time to make sure that everything was all right.

Three months later he was seen again. He said that he felt well and had no problems. He admitted to a drink 'about every week'. On one occasion a relative visited from Moscow with some 'special vodka' and he felt he 'had to drink a few glasses'. He was strongly advised to abstain completely but said this was not necessary as he was 'fully in control'. Mr Pillay was discharged from the clinic but was told that he could refer himself back if any problems arose.

During both interviews Mr Pillay's mental state was similar to that of the first interview, apart from a more marked insistence on his part that there was no longer a problem. By insisting there was no problem he made it difficult to explore further any facet of his life, whatever the emphasis chosen. The frame of reference of the interviews was shifted to that of a confirmation that all was well, rather than an exploration of what could be done to help. Any suggestion that there might be a problem or questions that might have hinted a problem was suspected were made to appear somehow impertinent. The psychiatrist decided to respect Mr Pillay's integrity and hoped that a sufficiently good engagement was made to enable him to return for help if this should prove necessary.

Four months later, Mr Pillay referred himself back to the clinic. He said, 'I had a few drinks and then went berserk.' He felt ill and described visual hallucinations of 'hideous animals'. A marked tremor was evident and he was very apprehensive. Mr Pillay, however, was not confused, and he was normally orientated in time and place. He was admitted to a psychiatric hospital with a diagnosis of 'acute alcoholic hallucinosis'.

Mr Pillay was an inpatient for four weeks. A physical examination performed on admission showed an enlarged, tender liver and a definite impairment of sensation below the ankles, but normal ankle reflexes. Investigations revealed abnormal liver function tests (gamma GT 66 IU/L; AST 44 IU/L). Alcohol withdrawal was covered with a chlordiazepoxide regime and in addition he was given multivitamin supplements. On the ward he was observed to be a quiet, shy man who never initiated conversations with others. Very little further information about his past history was elicited although he later admitted to drinking half a bottle of vodka per day for a few weeks before admission. He was noted to have no visitors. After two weeks in hospital he slipped out on a number of occasions and admitted to having had 'a few drinks'.

He was discharged from hospital much improved in his physical and mental state and was to be followed up in the outpatient department. However, he attended only once. On that occasion he claimed he was well and no longer drinking. His attitude was very similar to the one he had shown when first seen. There were no abnormalities on physical examination.

Mr Pillay did not keep his next appointment. Five months later, a work colleague brought Mr Pillay to the Accident and Emergency Department of the hospital. He smelt of alcohol, was tremulous, ataxic and disorientated, and appeared to be hallucinating. He was again admitted to hospital and again withdrawn from alcohol. A diagnosis of delirium tremens was made. A week after admission he developed an episode of acute pancreatitis which required emergency treatment but from which he recovered without incident. When he was more settled he was a little more forthcoming than previously. Following his previous admission to hospital he had struck up a relationship with a 24-year-old girl who suffered from a chronic and severe obsessive-compulsive disorder. He had met her on the ward. She was a shy, anxious girl whose psychological development had been disastrously interrupted by her severe symptoms and long periods of hospitalization from the age of 16. Mr Pillay said they had become engaged but then, after going to the cinema together and seeing a film with a strong sexual content, his fiancée had broken off their relationship. This was about six weeks before his admission and he had been drinking a bottle of vodka daily since then. Mr Pillay did not express anger towards his ex-fiancée but to a girlfriend of hers, also a patient, whom he accused of being jealous and at the same time prejudiced against him because he was an immigrant. Mr Pillay also talked of being lonely and of his friends being heavy drinkers. He had lost contact with those who were not. He was also seeing much less of his sister.

During this admission Mr Pillay was considered to be significantly depressed and he was treated with sertraline, 50mg a day. This had no effect on his mood. Just before his discharge from hospital, after seven weeks as an inpatient, he was suspected of drinking again. He had no visitors during this admission.

Mr Pillay failed to attend for follow-up after his discharge. Within four months he was readmitted with delirium tremens ushered in by an epileptic fit. He was disorientated and had auditory and visual hallucinations. Shortly before he had been attacked and robbed in the street by some youths. Liver function tests were again abnormal (gamma GT 80 IU/L). On neurological examination there was a definite impairment of sensation below the mid-calf level and ankle jerks were absent. Clinical cognitive testing following recovery from the acute confusional state showed no abnormality. Detailed psychometric tests were not, however, performed. This time, after a period of 'drying out', he was referred to a day hospital. He attended for a month and went to most of the prescribed activities, although he mixed poorly with the other patients. Most sessions with the registrar responsible for his care were centred around his broken engagement, which had a profound effect on his already shaky self-confidence. During weekends at home he had no social support and he lapsed into drinking. He was encouraged to attend AA meetings, which he did only sporadically, and another course of antidepressant medication failed to improve his mood. There were no signs of peripheral neuropathy on discharge and his gamma GT levels again fell to within the normal range. When he finally returned to work he was informed that he would lose his job if his drinking continued. He moved out of his flat and took a room with a Mauritian family.

For three months following his discharge Mr Pillay attended regularly as an outpatient. He denied that he was drinking but it was strongly suspected that he was. He attended AA irregularly. He was always polite and deferential in his manner but again revealed very little about himself. Nothing new emerged about his past life, nor was it ever clear what he was feeling during the sessions. He maintained that all was going well and he seemed to be gaining a measure of new support from the family with whom he was living. He contributed to the house by doing some redecorating and took some pride in this. An offer of Antabuse, to see whether it would help him avoid drinking, was rejected. He eventually lapsed from follow-up again.

## Reassessment

As predicted, Mr Pillay's drinking has continued with serious consequences. This gloomy situation creates a sense of fatalism and hopelessness, which although frequently realistic, inhibits exploring alternative potential areas of help.

### Diagnosis

Mr Pillay has continued to show dependence on alcohol with a series of syndromes of alcohol withdrawal – generally delirium tremens, but on his second admission an acute hallucinosis in clear consciousness. There has been a marked deterioration in his social functioning and his job has been threatened. A number of other complications of alcohol abuse have been present – liver damage, peripheral neuropathy and an episode of acute pancreatitis. They have so far proved reversible. The pattern of drinking seems to be one of intermittent spells of very heavy consumption interspersed with periods of more controlled, lesser consumption. This is probably why, despite many years of drinking, physical complications have not been more in evidence.

## Aetiology

During the year or so since Mr Pillay first presented, there has been a great deal of evidence to confirm his social isolation and his difficulty in sustaining close relationships. No concern about him has ever been expressed to doctors by any friend or even his sister. He was never visited in hospital. He entered into a relationship with a young and very disabled girl, which looked doomed from the beginning. His expectation that it would result in a 'normal marriage' was grossly unrealistic. His reaction to their break-up showed a marked sensitivity to rejection and in addition he was unable to perceive its origins in their relationship but instead blamed someone else. He has remained secretive and has failed to establish anything more than a superficial relationship with his doctor.

## Further information

It is striking that an informant has never been seen. At first Mr Pillay refused, but after this the issue seems to have been entirely lost. Had it been raised again it is possible that he might have relented and that his sister could have been interviewed. Some information might have been obtained which could have proved helpful in understanding why he was so concerned to avoid talking about himself. This might have suggested a better strategy for reaching him. The issue of an informant was probably lost because doctors had given up on him and because they sensed his likely embarrassment were certain facts to emerge. The subject was a difficult one to broach with him and the cues he gave were to avoid it. It has meant, however, that he remains in many respects an enigma. A home visit could be organized by a social worker or community nurse. This might provide some useful information but it is unlikely that it will help to engage him in continued treatment.

## Management

Mr Pillay has never stated unequivocally that he wishes to stop drinking, and even during his inpatient treatment he used to slip out for some alcohol. Antidepressant medication has not improved his mood, and he has rejected the offer of Antabuse. A therapeutic alliance with the doctor has not been established, and he only attended Alcoholics Anonymous meetings sporadically.

Given his consistent failure to cooperate in any more than a superficial way, the only option is to wait and see what happens. Mr Pillay has shown some inclination to return to the hospital when he becomes very ill and it is hoped he will return again when the need arises. Perhaps some new information will emerge or he will change his attitude. Considerable pressure should be exerted on him to allow an independent informant, such as his sister or a colleague, to be seen.

Referral to a specialist alcohol service needs to be considered if he returns.

## Prognosis

This is very gloomy. It is likely that Mr Pillay will continue to drink, develop further physical and psychological complications and lose his job. His decline appears to be accelerating. Although there have been no intimations so far, the possibility of suicide should be considered, particularly if he were to lose his job. Perhaps a small hope resides in the support that he might be receiving from the family with whom he is now living.

## Postscript

No more was heard of Mr Pillay for about nine months. He was then readmitted with the help of a work colleague, again with delirium tremens. His case notes regarding this admission were interspersed with many comments concerning his lack of motivation to stop drinking. No new points emerged in the history. However, he had managed to hold down his job and was still living with the same family. It was arranged for him to be seen at a specialist alcohol treatment unit where he was finally admitted. In the three years following this he never reappeared at his district hospital but it is known that he continued to hold his job.

# Chapter 8

# A Solicitor's Request

## Mr Loyola

### Presenting complaint

A phone call was received from a solicitor, asking for a psychiatric opinion on Mr Loyola who had been charged on two counts of criminal damage, and one of grievous bodily harm. Having ascertained that it was possible to see his client and prepare a report in good time for his next hearing, the psychiatrist asked the solicitor to send a letter, setting out the points on which he wished to have an opinion, and copies of any statements in his possession. Copies of 12 statements, a list of two exhibits, a charge sheet with a list of previous convictions (all prepared by the police) and a copy of Mr Loyola's statement to his solicitor were accordingly sent with the letter.

The statements were of three kinds: by complainants, by expert witnesses (a doctor and a telephone engineer), and by Mr Loyola, under caution to various police officers. Many of the statements were reports by different witnesses of the same incidents and, other than those of Mr Loyola, there was little variation between them. In fact they very often used exactly the same words. It was possible to build up a reasonable picture from them of the three alleged offences.

The first incident, leading to the charge of grievous bodily harm, occurred when Mr Loyola became involved in a feud between two families, the Porters and the Tanners. He, John Porter and one other youth went to Mr Tanner's home to exact retribution on one of the family's male members. Mr Loyola took the lead in this affair and got into an argument with Mrs Tanner on the doorstep, which led to him hitting her twice with a hammer. The youths then ran off leaving Mrs Tanner lapsing into unconsciousness and covered in blood. On admission to hospital that evening Mrs Tanner was reported by the house surgeon to be drowsy and disorientated and to have weakness of her left side, and an extensor left plantar reflex. There were injuries to her head and an abrasion over the lower thoracic spine. Four epileptic fits were observed shortly after admission but no radiological evidence of skull or spinal fracture was seen. She was treated with phenytoin and her condition resolved spontaneously over an eight-day admission. An EEG performed before discharge was normal, but she was advised to take prophylactic long-term phenytoin.

Four of the prosecution witnesses stated that Mr Loyola's assault was unprovoked. Mr Loyola stated, under caution, that he had attempted to hit Mr Tanner, was intercepted by Mrs Tanner who had kneed him in the groin, and that he had then 'cracked up' ('blacked out' to his solicitor) and 'started bashing away'. He was therefore pleading not guilty on the basis that he was defending himself against attack.

The second incident occurred about three weeks later when Mr Loyola had gone to the local social security office. He had asked to see a supervisor to request additional benefits, but he was told that, because of his previous aggressiveness, none of the staff would discuss this with him. The witnesses stated that Mr Loyola then began to shout, pulled a telephone off its wires and punched a clerk in the stomach, 'very lightly' according to the clerk, before leaving. A telephone engineer confirmed that the wires had been ripped from the telephone, and that the damage would cost £20 to repair. Mr Loyola intended to plead guilty to this offence, but described it as 'a joke'.

The third incident occurred when Mr Loyola was being questioned about the other two. He was put into a detention room, although he later claimed that he had warned the police that he would 'crack up' if he was confined. Some time later a police officer returned to the room and found that Mr Loyola had gouged out pieces of the door, using the leg of a chair that he had broken. The officer reported that Mr Loyola had given the reason, 'I just get so worked up.' Mr Loyola was pleading not guilty to this offence.

Mr Loyola had ten previous offences dealt with by juvenile courts between the ages of 14 and 16, including one for assault, several for carrying a weapon (a knife), and several for theft of motor cars. His only recorded previous conviction in an adult court was for driving whilst uninsured.

In his letter, the solicitor specifically asked about the following points:

- Given that his client developed 'claustrophobia' in confined spaces and had done so when held by the police for questioning, should he be held not to be criminally responsible for his destructive behaviour whilst in the cell, and hence not guilty?

- Could some other psychiatric reason be found to 'affect his criminal responsibility' for his other destructive behaviour (in which case his guilty plea might be reversed)?

- Although psychiatric factors (his 'black-out') could not diminish his criminal responsibility for the GBH charge ('but please confirm') could they be a mitigating factor, and should he be receiving treatment?

- In the penultimate paragraph of his letter the solicitor expressed his concern about his client's fits of temper which could be 'extremely dangerous', and over the telephone the doctor was told that his client had stated that he would kill someone if he was sent to prison and so separated from his mother who, he said, relied on him.

An outpatient appointment was made, for which Mr Loyola arrived slightly early with another young man. Very unusually, the reception staff rang to ask that the doctor see Mr Loyola with the minimum of delay because he was causing a disturbance. In itself, what he was doing – roaming round the waiting area, verbally accosting other patients and staff and talking loudly and boastfully to his friend – was little enough, but the staff were frightened of him. The psychiatrist decided to see him in a room with an alarm button and near to the nurses' station, and to start the interview with a general account of his background.

Mr Loyola had no clear complaints. He would one moment say that he was perfectly okay – 'I'm no nutter' – and then that his solicitor thought 'there must have been something wrong' for him to do what he did. He seemed to be in conflict about being thought to have any psychiatric problems: on the one hand the court might take a more lenient view if he had a psychiatric disorder, but on the other hand, he was unwilling to be considered in need of anyone's help.

The history was difficult to obtain although Mr Loyola became calmer when he was told that he could only be seen alone, not with his friend, and after the doctor wondered aloud whether Mr Loyola's restlessness was an expression of his fear of psychiatric hospitals.

He eventually gave the following account.

## Family history

Mr Loyola was the only child of a Spanish father aged 56 and an English mother aged 54. His father had been married and had children before leaving Spain to come to the United Kingdom, but nothing was known of this family. As long as Mr Loyola had known him, his father had been a heavy drinker and had had an explosive temper. Mr Loyola remembered from an early age his father hitting his mother and hearing his unfounded accusations of her infidelity. In more recent times Mr Loyola and his father had come to blows. There had been several occasions during his childhood when his father had 'disappeared'. One of these was for a year. Mr Loyola thought he had been living with other women during these periods. He had permanently left the family when Mr Loyola was 14. Mr Loyola had seen him occasionally at work in the subsequent two years, but he had not been heard of since.

Mr Loyola's mother had worked throughout his childhood and had usually been the breadwinner. Mr Loyola described her as a 'nervous wreck'. However, Mr Loyola also described himself as being very close to his mother, but said, 'I hate my father.'

## Personal history

Mr Loyola was born in hospital. He thought that his development had been normal and that he had been a healthy baby. He had lived throughout his life in a deprived area in a northern city. His mother had worked long hours when he was young and so after school he had been cared for by an elderly neighbour, about whom he could now remember little. At the age of six he had been run over by a car whilst on a pedestrian crossing and suffered a head injury. Mr Loyola dated his tempers from this incident, and said that subsequently he had often been in trouble at school for violence. This was usually directed at members of staff but also sometimes at other boys, who teased him and called him 'fatty'. He was expelled from two schools for violence. On the second occasion, when he was 14, he described coming upon his headmaster leaning out of a sash window which Mr Loyola forcibly closed, trapping the man by the neck and then belabouring him with blows and kicks. Subsequently he failed to settle at two other schools, would not cooperate with a home tutor, and consequently failed to become proficient in either reading or writing. Mr Loyola worked from the age of 16 to 17½ with the council road maintenance department, as did his father, but estimated that he had subsequently had about 30 jobs, which had each ended after rows with his bosses. Currently he and a partner planned to set up their own painting and decorating business, having attended an evening class in 'do-it-yourself'. He would not discuss these plans and no assessment could be made of how realistic they were. Mr Loyola had always lived at home with his mother. He had no current regular girlfriend and had broken up with the girlfriend he had had since he was 16, because she was getting too serious. Although Mr Loyola said that he had frequent sexual relationships he was unwilling to discuss these, or any other aspects of his sexuality.

Mr Loyola was well known in his area, and did not lack for companions. However, he appeared to have few, if any, close relationships, other than his stated closeness to his mother. Mr Loyola's main interests were his car and karate. He visited the gymnasium four days a week, although the training programme had proved 'too much like hard work' for him to try and obtain a black belt. He was also a regular pub-goer and drank beer heavily on Friday and Saturday nights. He never drank alone, nor anywhere else but the pub, and had never experienced withdrawal symptoms. About 18 months before, he used stimulants for a short while, which he had bought from 'mates at the pub', but had found they made him 'too edgy'.

Mr Loyola had controlled the course of the interview so far, but further relevant information had to be obtained by more direct questioning, although it seemed likely he would experience this as pressure on him. He had previously been very restless and the interviewer felt that there was a constant danger that he would suddenly walk out of the interview. It also seemed unlikely that Mr Loyola could be relied upon to attend a second interview.

It was therefore expedient to obtain the information that would enable the lawyer's questions to be answered as economically as possible. In order to do this, the interviewer decided to reconsider what he had observed of Mr Loyola's mental state, and then make a preliminary formulation.

## Mental state examination

### Appearance and general behaviour

Mr Loyola was a plump man who looked younger than his age. He was rather restless throughout the interview, getting more so as it progressed.

### Speech

His speech was rapid and loaded with swear words. He referred constantly to 'Paki-bashing', fights with 'the Bill' (the police) and his own physical strength and fighting ability. He said at one point to the interviewer, 'I could easily take you on.' The form of his speech was normal.

### Mood

Mr Loyola described himself as being depressed all the time and 'totally fed up', but he did not look sad.

### Thought content

He was very worried about the possibility of going to prison.

*Abnormal beliefs and interpretations of events*

None had been detected.

*Abnormal experiences*

None were alluded to, or apparent at the interview.

*Cognitive state*

His memory and concentration appeared to be good.

## Preliminary assessment

Mr Loyola is a 21-year-old inner city resident with an over-worked mother who was probably usually too tired to be much of a parent to him, and a heavy drinking, quick-tempered father who never made an enduring relationship with either his wife or his son. He has had a history of temper tantrums stretching back into childhood when he had a head injury. He has been charged with three offences of violence about which his solicitor would like an opinion and the formulation will need to concentrate on these issues. Since there is a constant threat that the interview will end suddenly, the psychiatrist will have to decide whether Mr Loyola has a psychiatric illness.

*Diagnosis*

The most immediate consideration is whether Mr Loyola's personality has changed recently. If so, this might indicate that Mr Loyola has recently developed a psychiatric illness. Mr Loyola has committed three offences within a short period and after two years during which he has not been convicted of an offence. However, a change in his behaviour alone is a weaker indication of disorder and may be due to a change in his circumstances.

There are few symptoms and signs, independent of his behaviour, to suggest a psychiatric illness. There is no suggestion at all of a psychosis. Mr Loyola does complain of feeling depressed and also of panic in confined spaces. These symptoms, if they are recent, may indicate a depressive disorder or an anxiety neurosis, both of which may increase irritability and predispose to violence. Mr Loyola is also a heavy drinker, and the possibility of alcohol dependence leading to chronic intoxication and consequent abnormally impulsive or explosive behaviour needs to be considered.

The next consideration is whether Mr Loyola has a personality disorder. This is a difficult judgement to make, particularly in a patient who denies being in need of help but wants a court report and who may therefore give a very biased account of himself. Our experience has been that it is useful to consider three independent criteria and that all of them should be satisfied if a diagnosis of personality disorder is to be made. There should be evidence of some particular socially deviant behaviour, or a cluster of related behaviours, which are habitual and not under Mr Loyola's control. By itself, this may indicate only that Mr Loyola belongs to a sub-group whose culture admits of such behaviour. There should, therefore, also be evidence that these have adversely affected Mr Loyola's capacity to work or to gain satisfaction in social relationships. Finally, the features of Mr Loyola's personality should correspond to common descriptions of personality disorder. This last criterion has the following advantages: it can be made more explicit than the second criterion; in some cases it suggests the presence of other symptoms or signs which can be searched for; and it may be helpful in guiding management. The information obtained so far suggests that all three criteria are likely to be met, but a diagnosis of personality disorder (the type of psychiatric disorder relevant to Mr Loyola's case) cannot be made until evidence of socially deviant (in Mr Loyola's case, aggressive) behaviour is obtained, other than that which has led to the report being requested.

Two categories of personality disorder may be applicable to Mr Loyola. The first is personality disorder with antisocial manifestations (ICD10), or dissocial personality disorder (DSMIV). This would be consistent with Mr Loyola's lack of close relationships (although not his avowed close attachment to his mother), with his history in childhood of aggressive behaviour, and with his non-aggressive misbehaviour. However, it excludes emotionally unstable personality disorder (ICD10), a term best reserved for explosive outbursts that the affected person regrets and usually attempts, although often without success, to control. Frequently patients fulfil criteria for more than one type of personality disorder.

*Aetiology*

Although it is too early to consider these in detail, certain factors suggest themselves for direct enquiry.

A closed head injury, such as Mr Loyola suffered at the age of six, is associated with an increased risk of emotional or conduct disorders, especially irritability. These disorders may be the only detectable sequelae, or there may also be signs and symptoms of brain damage, possibly including epilepsy.

Brain damage in children may be the cause of persistent learning difficulties leading to failure at school, itself a contributor to adolescent conduct disorder.

Epilepsy, especially temporal lobe epilepsy, is itself associated with irritability. 'Automatic' violence may occur during the state of clouding of consciousness pre-ictally, post-ictally or actually whilst paroxysmal electrical activity occurs in the brain. By definition this behaviour is not purposeful but onlookers may, rarely, have difficulty in appreciating the behavioural impairment. Irritability is also commoner in epileptic patients between fits, sometimes in association with mild electrophysiological disturbance, which in some patients builds up over time until the epileptic threshold is reached.

Alcoholic intoxication is highly associated with all crimes of violence, but is particularly likely to predispose to outbursts in patients with a history of head injury.

Developmental factors contributing to a possible personality disorder are plentiful in Mr Loyola's history. His father's violent and antisocial behaviour, his mother's neglect, the serious marital and familial conflict, the lack of firm and consistent sanctions, poor relationships with his peers and his problems at school are all associated with truancy, stealing and other conduct disorders in childhood and with personality disorder in adulthood.

*Further information*

Further information relevant to diagnosis needs to be obtained. Is there evidence of epilepsy? Is there evidence of irritability due to a specific, treatable disorder such as depression, or to a specific handicap such as brain damage? More information needs to be obtained about the incidents themselves, particularly about Mr Loyola's intentions and feelings beforehand, about his attitude now, and about the part played by disinhibiting factors such as alcohol, or bravado.

Further information about Mr Loyola's personality is also needed, particularly about its development, about his behaviour towards other people close to him, and about his interests and habits. There are also pointers to areas of enquiry relevant to management. First, Mr Loyola seems to have had many fewer convictions between 16 and 20 than he had between 14 and 16. Were there factors operating then which would be relevant to the prevention of offences in the future? Second, a probation order will almost certainly be one of the recommendations that the psychiatrist will consider. It is therefore worthwhile enquiring specifically whether Mr Loyola has been on probation, something which may not be apparent even from extensive prosecution statements and, if so, how useful his relationship with a probation officer was to him. Three forensic questions, which will affect sentencing, have also been posed. Did claustrophobic panic affect his responsibility for the criminal damage? Is there any significance in his report of a 'black-out' when he committed the assault? Is his condition amenable to treatment? In order to answer these, Mr Loyola's mother should be interviewed, and previous psychiatric records obtained, and the probation service contacted. Special investigations, such as neuropsychological assessment focused on determining intelligence level and impulsivity, and MRI and EEG should be considered when this other information is available.

*Management*

Although not enough information is available for a plan of long-term management to be made, the conduct of the rest of the interview is also an aspect of management. The most important consideration appears to be that Mr Loyola feels that his coming to see a psychiatrist has wounded his pride. One way of reducing his anger about this (which might otherwise prompt him to cease to cooperate altogether) is to allow him to tell his story in his own way, and for the interviewer to reduce control over the progression of the interview to the minimum consistent with obtaining necessary information. It would also be important to balance lines of enquiry about his deficiencies, for example his difficulty in reading and writing, with opportunity for him to expatiate on his sources of self-esteem.

### Prognosis

This appears to be poor, at this stage. However, more information is required, as outlined above, in order to discuss this.

### Further details

The interview was completed, but Mr Loyola refused to attend again, either for a follow-up interview or for further investigations. Mrs Loyola, his mother, was interviewed on another occasion. Although it proved that Mr Loyola had seen a psychiatrist on at least two previous occasions, the notes could not be obtained as the hospital where they were kept had been closed, and the records destroyed. However, a psychiatrist who had seen Mr Loyola and his family when he was 12 was contacted, and remembered something of his impressions. It was discovered that the court had ordered psychiatric and social enquiry reports in relation to the charges. The psychiatric report was not forthcoming because although Mr Loyola had attended to see the psychiatrist, the latter had failed to arrive within the half-hour that Mr Loyola had been prepared to wait. However, a copy of the social enquiry report was obtained. This further information, when collated, was as follows.

### Family history

Mrs Loyola confirmed that Mr Loyola senior had been extremely violent, and also jealous. They had never married, and she was unsure whether her son knew of this. She said that as her son grew up, he had become increasingly like his father.

## The offences

Mr Loyola thought that both of his acts of criminal damage were to some extent justified. In the case of the social security office, he felt that he had been unfairly treated, as the damage to the telephone was really too minor for consideration. He had no conception of the frightening effect of his rage on others. He also felt unrepentant for the damage to the detention room as he warned the police officer who took him to the room that he 'cracked up' in confined spaces, and because they had kept him waiting for an hour instead of the 20 minutes that they had said. Mr Loyola had not been drinking before either of these incidents. Alcohol usually made him 'merry' and not irritable. He did feel that authority in general, and the police in particular, 'had it in for me'.

His assault on Mrs Tanner perturbed Mr Loyola more. He had not previously known the Tanner family, but was acquainted with one of the Porters. This man and his brother had seen Mr Loyola in a pub, and had told him that four Tanners had attacked Mrs Porter and had asked him to help them 'sort it out'. He had replied, 'I might as well.' On his way to the Tanners in his car he had stopped off at home to get a specially weighted length of wood, despite later claiming that he was not intending to fight but only to talk. Mr Loyola subsequently took the lead in the expedition and continued to do so even after the Porter brothers dropped out of the party. He told the psychiatrist that he would not have struck Mrs Tanner had she not hit him which, he stated, made him 'go blank and lash out'. He instructed his solicitor that he intended to plead 'not guilty' on grounds of self-defence for this reason. He remembered hitting Mrs Tanner and then running away to his car, which had been concealed. He said that afterwards he disposed of the length of wood by throwing it into someone's garden. He next went back to the pub, and then to a cafe where he got into a row with the owner and left without paying. Mr Loyola did not seem remorseful about the injury caused to Mrs Tanner, but did seem very frightened of going to prison. He said, 'I'll kill anyone who sends me up.'

## Personal history

*School*

Mr Loyola had first been suspended from school for biting and kicking at the age of five, shortly after his father had left his mother. His mother had not been concerned about her son's behaviour, saying that it 'was a natural thing when they start school'. His education had subsequently been disrupted. He had failed to get into the army because of his 'poor maths'.

*Work*

Mr Loyola had lost a labouring job which had lasted a month about one month before the incident with Mrs Tanner, and he had not worked since.

## Forensic history

Mrs Loyola reported that her son had first been in trouble with the police at the age of 12. Although a list of Mr Loyola's previous offences was provided by the police, it emerged that this was incomplete and that several driving offences (connected with his continued use of his car after his licence had been suspended) were still outstanding.

Mr Loyola had been on probation for two years at the time of the offence. He had avoided contact with his probation officer, and resented his supervision. He did not feel that he had benefited from being on probation.

## Previous medical and psychiatric history

Mr Loyola had been knocked down on a pedestrian crossing at the age of six and suffered a head injury as already mentioned. Mr Loyola thought that he had been in hospital for one week after this and his mother thought that he had been unconscious for two days. Neither was absolutely sure. (It was too long in the past to assess his amnesia.) His mother had been awarded £150 compensation on his behalf.

Suspension from school made it impossible for any learning difficulty to be assessed at that time, but he had learnt to read simple words as already noted.

Mr Loyola had never had a fit or a faint. He could remember no deja-vu experiences and had never been depersonalized or experienced derealization. He said that once his violence was 'set off' he did not know that he was doing it but could recall afterwards what had happened. His description was more like a description of losing control, rather than an alteration of consciousness.

Mr Loyola had first seen a psychiatrist at about the age of five, having been referred by the school because of aggression. He attended intermittently for several years and his mother was seen regularly.

When Mr Loyola was 12 a psychiatrist made a domiciliary visit after Mr Loyola had attempted to stab his father with a knife. Although there were no written records, this psychiatrist remembered finding the whole family 'very disturbed' and had offered family therapy, which they did not accept. In fact, shortly after this Mr Loyola's father left the family.

For as long as he could remember, Mr Loyola had felt tense and angry when waiting or when feeling confined. He would not travel in tubes or buses for this reason. He was most comfortable driving in his own car, but always wound the windows down, even in winter. He disliked staying in one pub for any length of time, and could not sit through a film in a cinema. He could travel up to three floors in a lift but no more. Alcohol did not relieve these symptoms.

Mr Loyola was subject to overwhelming bouts of dysphoria, which he described as feeling 'empty'. These were worse when he stayed indoors or was alone for any length of time. They occurred once or twice a month. On these occasions he would shout at his mother, and had punched the walls, scattered cushions about and, sometimes, smashed furniture. He disliked watching television but enjoyed trying to mend mechanical or electrical things. However, if his repairs did not go well he would get into a tantrum with frustration and, at various times, he had smashed a television, a stereo and a video player.

Mr Loyola had never felt sad or tearful but often felt empty and 'fed up', as already noted. He had, he said, taken 'loads of overdoses', including one a month before the assault, 'because I had no money'. Usually these 'overdoses' were of his mother's diazepam. He had never had a definite intention to kill himself, and the overdoses usually occurred during an episode of dysphoria. He had once jumped in front of a bus and, the day before the interview, had been playing with live detonators, one of which exploded, burning his hand.

## Previous personality

Since childhood Mr Loyola had an explosive temper that he made little attempt to control. In adolescence this had become incorporated into a perception of himself as strong, powerful and masculine. He was unable to distinguish anxiety from anger. His self-esteem was easily bruised and he blamed others for anything that went wrong. He was intolerant of all authority, such as the police, but he also tended to glorify the violent side of the latter's work. He was racially prejudiced and described attacking 'niggers' and 'Pakis' both verbally and physically.

His mother said that he was 'easily led'. Mr Loyola had many acquaintances but no close friends. His mother described him as being very close to her but also reported that he had punched her on occasions.

Mr Loyola had had no close relationships with the possible exception of his mother and one girlfriend. He did, however, seem to attract male companions of his own age. Without constant companionship and activity he was subject to the bouts of dysphoria already mentioned.

## Physical examination

This was not performed.

## Mental state examination

*Appearance, general behaviour and speech*

This was as already described.

*Mood*

Mr Loyola's predominant mood continued to appear to be one of tension rather than sadness or unhappiness. He denied ever having felt anxious or fearful. He had a long-standing difficulty in getting off to sleep, but did not wake early. His appetite was good although food did not 'taste of much' to him. There had been no recent change in his concentration, memory, energy or libido.

### Thought content

He was hopeful about his future, as long as he could avoid going to prison. Mr Loyola worried about prison, but did not otherwise ruminate.

### Abnormal beliefs and interpretations of events

He had always been quick to assume that people were staring at him in the street or that casual remarks referred especially to him but was able to accept that he could not be sure that this was so. He was not deluded. He believed that he was well known to the police and that they victimized him.

### Abnormal experiences

When asked about hallucinations Mr Loyola remembered that as a child he had heard 'a man's voice shouting' when there was no one present and had thought he was 'going mad'. This had not recurred and he recounted no other abnormal experiences.

### Orientation

This was normal.

### Cognitive state

His attention and concentration were good, despite his physical restlessness. His memory was also good, and his dating of events relating to the offences, for example, matched closely that of the statements. Mr Loyola's grasp and rapidity of thought suggested that he was of normal to superior intelligence.

### Self-appraisal

Mr Loyola did not consider himself ill, or likely to benefit from psychiatric care.

## Reassessment

It is now possible to reformulate Mr Loyola's problems in order to answer the lawyer's questions.

*Diagnosis*

Mr Loyola lacks close social relationships and has failed to establish himself in steady work, despite over 30 attempts to do so, because of repeated uncontrolled explosions of rage. These have also led to his being banned from a social security office. He has failed to obtain a court-ordered psychiatric report because he refused to wait more than half an hour to see the psychiatrist.

Mr Loyola has had serious temper tantrums since he was five, when they led to referral to a psychiatrist. They caused him to be suspended from school on at least two occasions, once after a serious and unprovoked attack on a headmaster when he trapped the man's head in a sash window and then kicked him repeatedly. Recently he has smashed valuable articles at home in temper, and also punched his mother. Mr Loyola's episodes of dysphoria may also be related to his tantrums because, according to his mother, he usually dealt with them by trying to get into a quarrel with her. A possible connection may be that Mr Loyola feels 'empty' and 'fed up' when frustrated but unable to attack someone or something else who he feels is to blame.

There is also other evidence of repeated antisocial behaviour. Mr Loyola regularly played truant from school, and had first been involved with the police at the age of 12. He had many appearances in juvenile court for both theft and assault. Picking fights with 'Pakis' was one of Mr Loyola's main stated interests. He characteristically adopted a belligerent air with anyone whom he took to be an authority figure, as evinced by his behaviour during the interview.

Mr Loyola does not recognize that he has a problem with his behaviour, nor is his antisocial behaviour entirely due to attacks of rage. Mr Loyola therefore meets the criteria of a personality disorder with dyssocial or antisocial manifestations rather than of an explosive personality disorder. There is convincing evidence that Mr Loyola has a personality disorder since all three criteria of personality disorder are met: habitual undesirable behaviour, which is antisocial in Mr Loyola's case, and which results in social dysfunction and is characteristic of a recognized personality type.

Mr Loyola's personality is not so severely disordered, nor the incidence of serious violence so frequent that the possibility of other contributory psychiatric factors can be excluded without further consideration. One candidate already considered in the initial formulation is epilepsy. However, both Mr Loyola and his mother stated that he had never had an unexplained fit or a faint. The violent episodes are not typical of either psychomotor seizures or epileptic automatism: Mr Loyola's behaviour is purposive during them rather than stereotyped, he has some memory of what happens, and he is capable of rational conversation during his outbursts.

Another possibility is that Mr Loyola has had an affective disorder that may have contributed to his instability and explosiveness.

Depression may be more difficult to diagnose in a patient with an antisocial personality. Some psychiatrists would extend the term widely in order to explain antisocial behaviour. However, in preparing a report for the Court it is wisest to base the diagnosis on such typical signs and symptoms of depressive disorder that there are, independent of the offence. Mr Loyola describes himself as 'depressed' and 'totally fed up' and said he was so one month before the assault when he took an overdose. Mr Loyola has deliberately harmed himself on several previous occasions over many years. His feeling of being 'fed up' was usually short-lived, although it may have become more prolonged since the offences, because of his fear of going to prison. He is not hopeless about the future, and has expansive plans to start his own business. He shows none of the 'biological' features of depression: there has been no change in his appetite and weight, he does not wake early in the morning, his concentration and memory are both unimpaired, he is continuing with his usual interests and he can enjoy himself. A diagnosis of depression cannot therefore be sustained.

The possibility of an anxiety state is suggested by Mr Loyola's dysphoria and his difficulty in falling asleep (a symptom often found in anxiety states, but not specific to them). Mr Loyola confuses anxiety and anger, making it difficult to assess whether his level of anxiety is pathological. However, he does not experience his anger as 'suffering', he does not consider himself disabled by it, and he has no somatic symptoms, such as palpitations or tremor. This makes the diagnosis of anxiety neurosis inappropriate.

Although Mr Loyola is not suffering from an affective disorder, it could still be argued that he was in a temporary state of unusual irritability. For example he could have been under unusual stress after losing his job. However, the diagnosis of personality disorder does not exclude such fluctuations, and the diagnosis of acute stress reaction or adjustment disorder is not appropriate, because Mr Loyola's behaviour has not changed in kind, although it may have in intensity, as a result of the stress. Although Mr Loyola could not distinguish between anxiety and anger, he did distinguish panic from anger, describing it as 'cracking up', and was clear that this only occurred in specific situations, particularly confinement. Both Mr Loyola and his lawyer referred to this as claustrophobia. Mr Loyola's difficulty in using public transport, his avoidance of lifts and his avoidance of travelling in a car with the windows shut strongly suggest that he does have a significant disorder as they suggest. Claustrophobia may be present alone as a specific phobia or may be part of a wider agoraphobic syndrome when it is associated with a fear of unfamiliar places or situations. This fear is often greater with greater distance from home and is reduced in company. It may be significant that Mr Loyola brought someone with him to travel across London to see the psychiatrist. Phobic neuroses of this kind are in our experience commoner in patients with antisocial personality disorder and may be often related to the need to feel constantly in control.

*Aetiology*

The aetiology of personality disorder is controversial. It is almost certainly multifactorial. The following factors have probably contributed in Mr Loyola's case: neurological, imitative, developmental, social and contingent. Each of these suggests different management strategies.

### NEUROLOGICAL

Mr Loyola's head injury in childhood may, if sufficiently serious, have left him with an increased tendency to attacks of rage. However, this cannot be the sole cause as explosiveness is only one aspect of Mr Loyola's violence, which anyway first began when he was five, before his head injury.

### IMITATIVE

Mrs Loyola felt that her son had become 'more and more like her husband' in his attitudes and behaviour. This is unlikely to be attributable to heredity, which determines the transmission of much more elementary characteristics, but it can be explained by Mr Loyola's unconscious imitation of his father, whose behaviour and temperament were very similar to Mr Loyola's own.

### DEVELOPMENTAL

Mr Loyola has never developed an inner world of feeling, and therefore has difficulty in reflecting on or modifying his immediate emotional responses. As a result Mr Loyola lacks inner resources of self-esteem, and therefore depends heavily on the esteem of others. This may be one explanation of the apparent contradiction between his view that his behaviour is simply a reaction to others, and other people's experiences of him as being very controlling. Not enough is known of Mr Loyola's early relationship with his mother to pinpoint the origins of these developmental difficulties, although Mr Loyola was a 'latch-key' child from an early age, since Mrs Loyola returned to full-time work in his infancy.

### SOCIAL

Mr Loyola's standing among his peers was apparently enhanced rather than damaged by his antisocial behaviour. It is noteworthy that the targets that he usually chose (such as immigrants and the police) could be seen as 'out-groups', upon whom assault might be more socially acceptable to his peers. Although this is not applicable to the present assault, it was committed during a vendetta between two feuding families, and Mr Loyola excused his involvement in it on the grounds that he was righting a wrong.

CONTINGENT

It is often argued that violent behaviour is rewarded, and therefore sustained. However, apart from inflating his self-image, there is little evidence that Mr Loyola's behaviour is substantively rewarding. In fact, there are many occasions when Mr Loyola has suffered from his aggressive outbursts – for example when he has smashed valuable household items that would be expensive to replace, like a motorbike or a hi-fi.

Three of the aetiological factors – social, developmental and imitative – are likely, on the basis of clinical experience, to be particularly important in the genesis of Mr Loyola's antisocial behaviour. Their relative importance can only be established by observing the effect of changing one or other of them during his future management. Some historical information about the effects of changed social expectations is available inasmuch as Mr Loyola's frequency of offences fell whilst he had a steady girlfriend. He himself attributed this to her stabilizing influence.

*Further information*

A neurological examination and an EEG would be desirable, but Mr Loyola's refusal to re-attend precludes them. It is unlikely that a definite neurological abnormality would be found.

The attitude of the probation service to a probation order should be explored.

*Management*

If Mr Loyola was concerned to reduce his situational anxiety, it is likely that he could be considerably helped by a behavioural technique, such as desensitization or reciprocal inhibition. He is, however, less likely to respond to a treatment based on relaxation than someone whose fear of loss of control is not so great. There is no simple treatment for Mr Loyola's personality disorder, but regular contact with a sympathetic and skilled professional may allow early detection of increased stress and consequently reduce the likelihood of violence. However, his personality is such that he easily feels slighted, is intolerant of frustration, and copes with many situations by exploding into a rage. The chances of developing a therapeutic alliance with Mr Loyola are therefore low.

Mr Loyola does appear to suffer from a moderate degree of claustrophobia, which may have caused him to panic when enclosed in the detention room. He said that he damaged the door of the detention room in his desperate attempt to get out, and it is true that panic may lead to individuals with a phobia taking extreme steps to escape from the feared situation.

The solicitor also raised the question of Mr Loyola's plea. This is not usually a psychiatric matter but he may have been referring to Mr Loyola's 'intent'. This is a difficult and technical legal question rather than a psychiatric one. It is best to give the Court the relevant psychiatric evidence without further comment although, as there has been a suggestion of a 'black-out' that may suggest automatism to the Court, the following statement could also be added: 'There is no evidence that Mr Loyola was unaware of the nature of his actions during any of the three incidents.'

The recommendations about treatment should mention the possibility of treatment as part of a probation order. However, it should also be stated that the probation services must agree that an order is feasible. As it seems unlikely that Mr Loyola would attend, even if psychiatric treatment were a condition of probation, a probation order cannot be recommended.

Mr Loyola might benefit from treatment, support and supervision but only on a voluntary basis, which, as already discussed, he is not prepared to accept. No specific recommendation about treatment can therefore be made to the Court.

*Prognosis*

Mr Loyola's prognosis will depend a great deal on his future social relationships. He may find a niche in a criminal fraternity, he may meet a strong, masculine but law-abiding figure whom he can imitate and then identify with, or he may continue to have difficulties in social relationships in which case he is likely to become increasingly vulnerable to depression or alcoholism with age.

Mr Loyola is likely to become less explosive with the passage of years but the risk of a repetition of serious violence will remain for some time in the future. A period of imprisonment seems likely either following the present offence, or in the future.

## Postscript

Shortly after a court report was completed, Mr Loyola was remanded in custody. His mother had 'phoned the police during a row with her son, asking them to "put him away"'. Police officers had then gone to the house to interview Mr Loyola, who had attacked them. He had been arrested and charged with threatening behaviour.

Mr Loyola was subsequently sentenced to one year's Borstal treatment, but further details could not be obtained.

*Chapter 9*

# Fear of Going Out

## *Mrs Reiss*

**Presenting complaint**

Mrs Reiss' general practitioner referred her to the psychiatric outpatient clinic because of her fears of going out alone. She was a 48-year-old married woman of Slovak origin and said these fears had been present for six years, and for the past two years she had not ventured from her home unescorted. Attempts to go out alone resulted in panic and a fear of collapsing or dying. Mrs Reiss was somewhat better when driving a car but she could not manage a journey lasting more than five minutes or so. Travelling on public transport was avoided, as were enclosed spaces such as lifts, escalators and crowded, public places. The onset of these symptoms was described as sudden. Immediately following an argument with her husband, Mrs Reiss set out to post a letter but before she could reach the post box she was overwhelmed with anxiety and dizziness and was forced to struggle back to her home. Her movements were drastically restricted after this episode, but three years before presentation she improved considerably and for almost a year, although uneasy, she was relatively unrestricted in her movements. However, her symptoms returned with even greater intensity two years before presentation and this followed the discovery that her sister had advanced carcinoma of the ovaries from which she died a few months later. The immediate precipitant of her relapse was again a row with her husband, after which she went out shopping, became panicky, and had to be brought home by a stranger.

Mrs Reiss said that she felt apprehensive before leaving her front door and after a few minutes in the street she would become panicky, dizzy and sweaty, and could feel her heart pounding. At this point she would turn back to avoid the development of a full-scale panic attack. When accompanied by her husband or by one of her children she felt uneasy but was able to enter crowded places for short periods of time. She could only shop in a small store and then only if accompanied. She could reach her restaurant from home only by car even though it was less than two miles away.

Mrs Reiss also complained of being depressed and of difficulties getting off to sleep. Two years previously she had developed hypertension and this was a major concern to her. Although her doctor had told her this was mild (BP 160/100) she could not be reassured. Another source of unhappiness was her weight. When she was 20 years old she weighed 48kg but with the birth of each of her children and finally, following a hysterectomy four years previously, it continued to rise to its current level of 92kg. Attempts to lose weight had been invariably unsuccessful.

## Family history

Mrs Reiss came from a Slovakian Jewish family and lost both of her parents during the war when she was 14 years old. Her father was deported to an unknown destination while her mother and the children were taken to a concentration camp. There, her mother and three of her siblings were killed.

The family was a very religious one and she remembered her parents as being gentle and indulgent.

Two sisters and three brothers survived the war, Mrs Reiss being the youngest. Two years previously her elder sister died at the age of 66 of an ovarian carcinoma. Two brothers aged 59 and 56 were living in Australia. Both were happily married but both suffered from hypertension. The remaining brother, who had lived in the USA, died eight months previously aged 49. He suffered from hypertension and developed 'water in the lungs'. Mrs Reiss last saw him two years previously.

There was no family history of mental illness.

## Personal history

Mrs Reiss was born in a small town in Slovakia. Her birth and development were unremarkable and her memories of childhood were happy ones. She tended to be a reserved, shy girl but could not recall any special childhood fears. She recalled a marked sensitivity about menstruation as a girl. Her menarche occurred when she was 11 and her first period occurred while she was in the classroom. She felt extremely ashamed and feared returning to school until she was finally persuaded to do so after about a week.

As Mrs Reiss found it distressing to talk about her experiences during the war, these were not explored in any detail. However, references to 'the camps' cropped up frequently during the interview.

Almost immediately after the war, when she was 17, she married a schoolteacher in her hometown. She bore three daughters in four years, now aged 30, 29 and 27. Five years after her marriage, her husband died of meningitis at the age of 26. She was left with few supports, no close family and worked as a shop assistant for the next five years.

At the age of 26 she managed, with considerable difficulty, to escape from Czechoslovakia and emigrated to Israel. There, she re-established contact with some distant relatives and worked on a kibbutz.

Three years later, aged 29, she married an Englishman, 15 years her senior, and soon after they and her three children settled in Manchester, England. They started a restaurant together which proved quite successful and in which she was working up to 18 hours a day at the time of her referral.

Mrs Reiss described her husband as a 'good husband and father' but made a number of references to his 'strictness' and 'unsteady' temperament. She said that he seemed to disapprove of many of her activities, such as driving a car. He also liked to have her near him even when this seemed unnecessary. Sexual relations had been infrequent for many years. Despite some quarrels she said that the marriage was a happy one.

Mrs Reiss' children were all happily married and living in the same city.

Mrs Reiss said that she had very little free time. Her main pleasure was in seeing her grandchildren. She enjoyed listening to music and she was thinking of writing her biography. She rarely went out with her husband and she said that this was in part because of her fear of crowded places. A cinema, for example, was out of the question. Apart from the family, Mrs Reiss had no close relationships. She said she had made no new friends since her marriage.

## Past medical history

Four years previously, Mrs Reiss had a hysterectomy following investigation for menorrhagia. She did not know the reason. Two years before, her doctor diagnosed hypertension and prescribed propranolol, 10mg daily. She said her blood pressure had been 160/100.

As described previously, Mrs Reiss' weight had risen without her ever being able to reduce it to its previous level. She attempted to diet most of the time, but stopped attending Weight Watchers because she developed panic attacks when faced with a group of strangers.

## Past psychiatric history

Mrs Reiss had never sought psychiatric help. Her doctor had, however, prescribed a variety of 'tranquillizers', none of which seemed to help. She had taken chlordiazepoxide for about nine months, up until three months before coming to the clinic. She said that she was very sensitive to medication and readily experienced many side effects, particularly dizziness.

## Previous personality

Mrs Reiss described herself as 'a quiet and sensitive' person who was upset by loud noises, particularly shouting. While being able to mix quite well with other people in a friendly but superficial manner she found it difficult, because of her reserved nature, to open up more and make deeper relationships. She preferred to keep her thoughts to herself. Most of her energies were put into her home and work.

## Mental state examination

*Appearance and general behaviour*

Mrs Reiss was a moderately obese, well-dressed, pleasant woman who found it difficult to talk about herself. She gave the impression that she was unused to doing so and commented that it was unusual for her to show her feelings. On a number of occasions she was apologetic: 'I'm keeping you a long time, I'm sorry.'

## Speech

She spoke with a marked European accent but her English was good.

## Mood

During most of the interview Mrs Reiss did not appear especially dejected. She was animated when she talked about her children and grandchildren and she was able to laugh appropriately. On a number of occasions, however, her spirits sagged noticeably and she was on the point of tears. This happened when she discussed the war, the death of her first husband, the death of her sister and, most markedly, the death of her brother eight months ago. With regard to the last, there was no indication of any difficulty in accepting his death, of self-blame, of hostility or of an abnormal preoccupation with his loss. The intensity of her reaction did not appear unusually severe. This was also the case with regard to the death of her sister.

During the interview Mrs Reiss tended to be anxious and fidgety. She said she often felt 'tense and miserable'. However, she did not feel hopeless about the future and said, 'One day everything will be OK.' Although she expressed a reluctance 'to bother my family' with her problems she was not self-reproachful. She had never entertained any suicidal ideas. There was some difficulty in getting off to sleep 'because my breathing is not right', but she was then usually able to sleep right through the night, although she often had nightmares about the war. Mrs Reiss' appetite was normal and she was able to concentrate and function well at her work. Somatic symptoms of anxiety were only present when she faced going out on her own.

## Thought content

Mrs Reiss described her fears of going out in considerable detail, but with little emotion.

An important theme that emerged during the interview was that of illness. Mrs Reiss worried a lot about illness in others and in herself. 'After the camps when you hear things, it's worse.' Thinking about her raised blood pressure made her frightened and she found it difficult to accept that it was only mildly elevated. Unpleasant, though only momentary, sensations in her head she tended to attribute to her hypertension. Dizziness, in particular, was feared. She admitted to ruminating for long periods on her health and she made many visits to her GP asking him for further tests. She said she was easily fatigued and had to force herself to keep going.

*Abnormal beliefs and interpretations of events*
None were elicited.

*Abnormal experiences*
None were elicited.

*Cognitive state*
There were no abnormalities on cognitive testing.

*Self-appraisal*
Mrs Reiss said she needed help with her fears and expressed the hope, which she half-recognized as unrealistic, that there might be a tablet which could remove them. She was reluctant to commit herself to a course of treatment without knowing all the details first and said she might have difficulty in getting time off work.

## Physical examination

This was not performed, apart from taking her blood pressure. This was 160/90.

## Interview with informant

Her daughter accompanied Mrs Reiss. The history as given by Mrs Reiss was confirmed in all its essential points.

Mrs Reiss' daughter described her as someone who tended to worry excessively and was easily upset by displays of temper in others, by illness and by death (even in people she did not know well) and by any reference to war. However, she was also capable of stubborn determination particularly in her management of the business. Rarely had Mrs Reiss revealed her innermost feelings to anyone in the family, although her loyalty to them was unstinting. Mrs Reiss had rarely talked about her wartime experiences and she could not be drawn into discussion about her life during this period. To others she invariably gave the impression of being a friendly and cheerful but 'aloof' person.

The daughter said her mother and stepfather's marriage was good, although her stepfather could be rather rigid in his views and was often temperamental. At these times her mother retreated and arguments were never sustained. Mr Reiss was unable to understand his wife's symptoms but seemed to accept them with little irritation. Mrs Reiss had virtually no social life outside her immediate family.

Mrs Reiss was very distressed after the deaths of her sister and then her brother but she surprised her daughter with the apparent normality of her grieving.

## Assessment

Mrs Reiss presents with a six-year history of fear of going out alone as well as some more specific fears of enclosed spaces and of escalators. She complains also of feeling miserable, of being overweight and of the state of her physical health.

However, these problems are overshadowed by the implied enormity of her experiences as a concentration camp victim. It is therefore important to consider how these experiences might be related to her current condition without using them as a blanket explanation.

## Diagnosis

Mrs Reiss is suffering from agoraphobia with panic disorder. Most of the typical features are present including extreme anxiety if she should leave her home or another 'secure' place unaccompanied. Public or crowded places are particularly feared. She has been virtually housebound for the past two years and is only able to venture out in the company of a trusted friend. Her fears are irrational and grossly disproportionate, and they lead to avoidance of the feared situations. More specific fears, like those she described of escalators, are also common in patients with this condition, as are experiences of depersonalization.

The major differential diagnosis in this case is between agoraphobia as a primary disorder and its development secondary to a depressive illness. The relationship between agoraphobic symptoms and depressed mood is complex. Depressive symptoms not amounting to a depressive illness are common in patients with agoraphobia. However, agoraphobic symptoms may appear for the first time in the context of a primary depressive illness. In these cases the typical symptoms of a depressive illness would be apparent. The agoraphobic symptoms follow the natural history of the underlying illness and usually remit with the depression. The course is therefore likely to be one of a single episode lasting six to nine months or an episodic one with recovery between fairly clear-cut relapses.

In Mrs Reiss' case there is an absence of typical depressive symptoms, such as guilt, hopelessness or diurnal variation of mood. There is also the long duration of the agoraphobic syndrome, notwithstanding a fairly long period of partial remission. These points argue strongly against a primary diagnosis of depressive illness.

An atypical feature in Mrs Reiss' situation is the relatively late onset of her agoraphobic symptoms at the age of 42. Agoraphobia as a primary disorder usually commences before the age of 35 years.

Another notable aspect of Mrs Reiss' presentation is her preoccupation with her physical health. Although in part understandable in view of her strong family history of hypertension, her concerns with her blood pressure seem excessive and could be termed 'hypochondriacal'. They appear disproportionate to her mildly elevated blood pressure, they are associated with an unusual attention to physical sensations and she cannot be reassured as to their true nature.

The agoraphobia does not, in Mrs Reiss' case, appear in the setting of prominent anxiety symptoms outside the feared situations. Her tendency to worry excessively is a personality characteristic rather than a new development suggesting a morbid process.

There are also two physical diagnoses, obesity and hypertension. Mrs Reiss is clearly substantially above the mean weight for someone of her age and although her blood pressure was normal in the clinic it had been raised on a number of occasions when she consulted her general practitioner.

*Aetiology*

Mrs Reiss has had a life of extraordinary pain and misfortune. Although it is tempting to attribute all her difficulties to this, an attempt should be made to link her problems more specifically to particular antecedents.

An outstanding feature of Mrs Reiss' history is her wartime experience involving losses in her family and incarceration in a concentration camp. People who have survived this exposure to overwhelming fear, grotesque deaths, helplessness, physical abuse and dehumanization are often left with a number of special vulnerabilities and Mrs Reiss gives evidence of some of these. She has an indelible 'death imprint' which has sensitized her to illness and death, especially in relatives and friends. This was probably due to the impossibility of mourning her dead relatives in the midst of an appalling struggle for survival. Her experience of devastating loss of life, family and community are associated with a basic insecurity, a lack of a sense of social belonging and the loss of a sense of continuity with the past. After the war Mrs Reiss married quickly and it is easy to imagine how important it must have been for her to recreate a family life. Her first husband then died, again in circumstances when mourning must have been difficult, due this time to the needs of her young children and the requirement to press on in difficult times. Mrs Reiss' movements between different countries and the absence of a stable home must have also contributed to a sense of rootlessness and it is noteworthy that her symptoms have the effect of keeping her in one 'secure' place, her home.

It is in this context that Mrs Reiss' present relationship with her husband must be considered. A strong and stable family unit is especially important to her. She has no close relationships outside her family, not in itself surprising in someone who has experienced so much hostility in the world and who might thus have a pervasive difficulty in trusting outsiders. Although Mrs Reiss said that her marriage was a good one she described sensitivity to her husband's outbreaks of temper. A direct precipitant of her illness was a quarrel with her husband and a major exacerbation after a period of improvement also directly followed another quarrel with him. One senses that Mrs Reiss' loyalty to her family is such that she is unlikely to speak critically of them to an outsider and that her family is so crucial to her sense of security that she would be likely to tolerate much from her husband that was not to her liking. It is perhaps surprising that Mr Reiss did not accompany his wife to the hospital in view of the long history and the handicapping nature of her disorder.

Of more recent events in Mrs Reiss' life, the deaths of her sister and then her brother stand out. Bearing in mind Mrs Reiss' sensitivity to illness and death it does not come as a surprise that her agoraphobic symptoms emerged more intensely following her sister's illness and death. One might have expected to find evidence of a morbid grief reaction following these deaths, but this seems not to have been the case. She is sad about these losses but appears to have come to terms with them. The development of hypertension also coincided with the exacerbation of Mrs Reiss' symptoms and is likely to have acted as yet another stressful experience.

Overall, then, a number of Mrs Reiss' past life experiences can be seen as shaping a predisposition to some kind of psychological disorder as well as possibly exacerbating and maintaining one. However, why it should have taken the form of an agoraphobic syndrome is not fully explicable in these terms. In Mrs Reiss' case we do not have the benefit of a full family history that might have revealed similar problems in other members. Mrs Reiss' sensitivity to her menarche and her anxiety about going to school suggest that she was a rather anxious child, but this is tentative. A past history of school refusal and of undue separation anxiety is common in patients with agoraphobia.

Mrs Reiss' phobic symptoms can be seen more directly as the outcome of a learning process. Fears can be learnt as a response to previously neutral stimuli by 'classical' conditioning. This is most readily apparent for simple fears of specific objects. However, generalization from the initial stimuli may occur and here an important role can be ascribed to the symbolic associations of the stimuli for the individual. This type of learning is enhanced when the subject is anxious or distressed. In Mrs Reiss' case, the initial fear reaction occurred when she was emotionally distraught following a row with her husband. It occurred when she was in the street alone where multiple stimuli were available for association. Symbolic meanings for her, of crowded places and being alone, could have related to past experiences of crowded camps. Whatever the process of the learning involved, an important mechanism in perpetuating the fear (its failure to 'extinguish' with time) is the avoidance of the feared situation. By leading to a reduction in anxiety, avoidance in fact reinforces the fear.

Some understanding of Mrs Reiss' hypochondriacal preoccupations can be gained from the history. There is a strong family history of hypertension leading, in her brother's case, to death. The physical abuses experienced by concentration camp inmates may be associated with later concerns over bodily integrity and the fear of permanent damage. There may be some confusion in Mrs Reiss' mind between the sensations of 'dizziness' which she attributes to her hypertension and the 'dizziness' which she experiences during episodes of anxiety that serve to intensify her self-absorption in her physical state. Her sensitivity to the 'side effects' of tablets may also reflect her heightened vigilance to somatic sensations.

Mrs Reiss' obesity seems linked to a combination of weight increase with age and particularly in response to childbirth and hysterectomy. It is not the juvenile onset type where constitutional factors play a more important role. Past experience of starvation during the war might have contributed by creating a special preoccupation with food and, through the association of thinness, with suffering. Mrs Reiss' work as a caterer means that she is constantly exposed to food and this makes dietary restriction very difficult.

*Further information*

Although sufficient information has been obtained for a diagnosis to be made, before treatment can proceed a more detailed account is necessary of Mrs Reiss' fears and the limitations that they place on her. A clinical psychologist experienced in making such an assessment could propose a systematic treatment strategy based on learning theory principles.

It is not clear why Mrs Reiss, in view of the chronicity of her illness, has presented for help at this particular time. It is possible that a recent change in her circumstances, such as her marriage, has upset a pre-existing balance.

We do not know Mr Reiss' attitude to her symptoms although he must have been affected by them. Mr Reiss may need to be involved in treatment either in a general encouraging role or more directly in supervising her treatment activities. If there are important tensions in the marriage that contribute to Mrs Reiss' illness it might prove valuable to have some joint sessions. Mr Reiss thus needs to be seen both as an informant and to assess his willingness to be involved in the treatment.

Mrs Reiss' general practitioner should be consulted for further information about her hypertension and also about the treatment he has offered for her fears and her response to it. The precise reason for Mrs Reiss' hysterectomy is worth ascertaining as in someone with hypochondriacal concerns it may turn out to have been the result of persistent requests for help rather than of clear indications for surgery.

*Management*

Two alternative psychological methods should be considered, as well as the possibility of medication.

The first approach is supportive psychotherapy. The aim would be to establish a special type of 'working relationship' with Mrs Reiss in which she would find support and some advice in her endeavours to overcome her disabilities. Factors that have contributed to her illness could be explored with her in the context of a safe and trusting relationship with the therapist. Improvement would be predicted as the result of Mrs Reiss' acquisition of an understanding of her symptoms as arising from the oper-

ation of psychological influences, together with the therapist's encouragement to extend her range of activities in feared situations. The focus of
treatment would not be primarily on her symptoms but on the psychological mechanisms she employs in dealing with such problems as illness,
death and loss.

The second method, systematic desensitization, would focus more
directly on Mrs Reiss' symptoms, assuming them to be a learnt,
maladaptive response to situations that are reinforced by avoidance. The
principles involved are regarded as the same as those involved in normal
learning and are applied in the treatment. The situations Mrs Reiss fears
would be carefully delineated, as would her usual behavioural responses to
them. Treatment would require that she change her behaviour in the feared
situations and this would depend on exposure to those situations rather
than avoidance. A strategy of exposure could be planned, usually in a series
of graded steps representing a hierarchy of situations, increasing in their
fear-inducing qualities as perceived by the patient. Mrs Reiss would then
be encouraged to work through this hierarchy, progressing to the next step
when she is able to feel relaxed at the previous one. Relaxation exercises
might prove helpful here. It is anticipated that her fears will become
extinguished as avoidance is overcome and she learns that catastrophe
does not ensue from exposure. In theory the relationship with the therapist
would be different with this approach in that he or she would be more
didactic and less concerned with discovering 'psychological meanings'.

Although in practice there is considerable overlap between these
strategies there is good reason in Mrs Reiss' case for emphasizing a
behavioural approach. Given her past experience and the observations
made during her interview, it is likely that she will find it difficult to
establish the sort of trusting relationship with a stranger in which she will
feel comfortable in disclosing her inner feelings and in discussing the
powerful experiences in her past. Her cooperation is more likely to be
gained with an approach that is more directly linked to her presenting
complaints. The treatment can be carried out by a psychiatrist or a clinical
specialist in the outpatient department.

An antidepressant can be helpful when depressive features are prominent. Although in Mrs Reiss' case there is no indication for this at present, it is worth bearing in mind for the future as an adjunctive measure.

In some patients even when depression is not prominent, panic attacks and phobic symptoms can be helped by an SSRI or by a tricyclic antidepressant, although improvement usually requires a number of months of treatment. Benzodiazepines may also be of value in reducing anxiety, in the shorter term, if taken before the patient enters her feared situations. However, this does not generally help the patient to overcome her fears when she is not on medication.

In Mrs Reiss' case, where a long history is in evidence, a more direct attack on her symptoms is preferable to a palliative approach with benzodiazepines. There are two further worries about prescribing a benzodiazepine in her case: first, she is very sensitive to the unwanted effects of medication and these may make her even more preoccupied with her physical state; second, because of the chronicity of her fears, she may become dependent. A trial of an SSRI antidepressant could be held in reserve if a behavioural-psychotherapeutic approach fails to bring about an improvement.

Mrs Reiss' blood pressure needs to be monitored and at present propranolol, although in small dosage, seems adequate to control it. Propranolol also has a direct anxiety-reducing effect but usually at a higher dosage than prescribed here.

At this stage Mrs Reiss' hypochondriacal concerns and her obesity are not the most important issues. If her anxiety can be reduced, her hypochondriacal fears may also lessen. The treatment of obesity is difficult at the best of times and this could be left for review at a later stage if she overcomes her fears of going out alone.

### Prognosis

As Mrs Reiss' agoraphobic symptoms have been present for six years, the likelihood of a complete and permanent recovery from these is slight. A full recovery with this condition is most likely when the symptoms have been present for less than a year.

However, of importance in assessing the prognosis is Mrs Reiss' pre-morbid adjustment. Although her life has been an extremely difficult one she has been able to make a good adjustment in a number of respects. Despite the loss of her first husband, for example, she has managed to make a second and durable marriage. She has shown much determination in overcoming major crises in the past and her ability to work has remained unimpaired. These personality strengths are important in preventing the development of the even more severe disablement that may occur with this disorder.

Mrs Reiss' willingness to become involved in treatment will also be an important contributor to the eventual outcome. Her motivation for change is a little doubtful, particularly as she has delayed her request for help for such a long time.

Overall, it seems likely that Mrs Reiss will continue to function socially at a reasonable level, but that unless she works very hard with her treatment, her symptoms will persist to a variable degree. The severity of her symptoms is likely to depend on the occurrence of significant life events to which she is particularly vulnerable – loss, illness and death. These are likely to lead to exacerbations.

## Further details

A clinical psychologist saw Mrs Reiss, who was accompanied by her daughter as Mr Reiss was away in the USA on a business trip.

The psychologist's report was as follows:

> A detailed assessment of Mrs Reiss' fears was made. There are two categories of situations that are anxiety provoking: her distance from home (or a safe place) alone; and situations associated with looking up or down (e.g. escalators in tube stations).

> Situations inducing the highest self-ratings of fear on a 0–5 scale are: shopping in the local shopping centre; walking more than 15 minutes from home; a bus journey of more than 15 minutes; travelling on the underground; and using an escalator.

> Situations giving lesser difficulty (rated 2–3) include crossing a main road, shopping in a local shop, sitting in a cinema, visiting the synagogue and driving more than five minutes from home.

Mrs Reiss' fear is diminished by being accompanied by a trusted person, using a shopping trolley, darkness, having a way open for a quick return home and thinking about something else (especially her grandchildren). Her fear is made worse by arguments with her husband, hearing bad news especially concerning illness or death and having to cross a main road.

At present she cannot walk unaccompanied more than three houses from her own home but she can drive for five minutes before having to turn back.

Mrs Reiss' daughter also provided some useful information about her husband's contribution. She described him having contradictory views about the problem. On the one hand he usually behaves as if the problem does not exist or that it is simply a matter of will power, on the other hand he often maintains that if his wife has this problem then she should not drive, go out, etc. He appears to be contributing to the problem to some extent by discouraging her from going out, thus reinforcing her avoidance of feared situations.

When we discussed the circumstances surrounding the onset of her disorder Mrs Reiss told me that her symptoms first began a few months after her daughter had married and left home. She was the last of her children to do so. It followed immediately after a quarrel with her husband when they were on their way home from an enjoyable evening out with a group of friends.

When we discussed treatment Mrs Reiss seemed surprisingly reluctant to cooperate. However, after some discussion with her daughter she agreed to 'give it a try'.

The general practitioner confirmed that Mrs Reiss' hypertension was first noted two years previously and that it had been 160/105 on a number of occasions. Although it was well controlled with medication Mrs Reiss was unable to be reassured about this. He had not been aware of the full extent of Mrs Reiss' phobic symptoms although he had recognized that she 'suffered from anxiety for many years'. Chlordiazepoxide, 10mg twice daily, had been prescribed for about nine months but this did not prove helpful. The hysterectomy had been performed for persistent menorrhagia caused by fibroids.

## Reassessment

The psychologist has confirmed the nature of Mrs Reiss' problem. However, she has also discovered new details about its onset and also how her relationship with Mr Reiss has contributed to the overall picture. The main focus now is on treatment.

### Diagnosis

This is unchanged.

### Aetiology

Some important new points have emerged. Mr Reiss' attitude to Mrs Reiss' disorder is problematical and he expresses ambivalent feelings about it. His behaviour looks as if it encourages the maintenance of her symptoms. A new version of the onset of Mrs Reiss' symptoms again places it in the context of a quarrel with her husband. She is very likely to have experienced her daughter's departure, in part, as a significant loss, due to the importance she invests in her family. It also meant that she was now alone with her husband and probably left to confront problems with him more directly. However, it is still unclear why Mrs Reiss presented at this time.

### Further information

It will be important to assess Mr Reiss' attitude at first hand.

### Management

A behavioural strategy has been offered by the psychologist to be carried through by her. This involves a programme of graded activity with practice sessions in the hospital and prescribed daily 'homework'. She will be helped to construct a hierarchy of fearful situations, in ascending order of anxiety, and will work on these between sessions. For example, the first session planned will focus on her ability to leave her home, by encouraging her to walk increasing distances, each time up to a point where she can manage her anxiety. Mrs Reiss will be instructed to keep a diary of all of her outings and to record the distance travelled and anxiety experienced.

*Prognosis*

Mrs Reiss' questionable motivation and Mr Reiss' apparent ambivalence might prove important limitations on progress.

## Further details

Mrs Reiss embarked on, and persisted with, the treatment planned with the psychologist. She was seen weekly for six weeks, then fortnightly for six sessions, then at monthly intervals.

The emphasis remained on desensitization 'in vivo'. For the first month Mrs Reiss cooperated well, although her homework tended to be unsystematic. She kept her record of outings diligently but suddenly recorded higher anxiety ratings than previously.

Mrs Reiss' deterioration appeared to be due to her husband's responses to her treatment. On his return from the USA he tended to disparage her gains and on one occasion said that anyone ought to be able to go out alone and that she ought to be able to do this without any help from the hospital. Mrs Reiss became extremely distressed about this and stopped practising. Several attempts to see Mr Reiss following this episode were unsuccessful. The next session was spent mainly in discussion of how she could deal with her husband's reaction and in devising ways in which praise from other family members could be maximized.

When the psychologist rang Mrs Reiss' home in order to change the next appointment her husband answered the phone. Mr Reiss seemed more helpful than the impression given by his wife. At one point he blamed himself for his wife's condition, stating that because of a heart attack and the medication he was prescribed, he was unable to give her 'enough love'. He said he often felt very depressed about himself. Mr Reiss was invited to attend the next session with his wife, but said that because of business pressures this would be unlikely.

For the next four weeks Mrs Reiss made considerable progress and was recording zero anxiety with 15-minute walks. She made two journeys on the underground and had used an escalator at a large shopping complex. However, over the following two weeks she again suffered a major setback, recording very high anxiety levels, stopping all practice and eventually retiring to her bed. During the next visit she complained that her husband distracted her when she was about to go out and gave her other jobs to do. Her general practitioner had increased the dose of propranolol and she felt this was making her dizzy. She had recently spoken to someone who had 'blacked-out' on similar medication and was distressed by this. She gave the impression that when she was ill her husband became more considerate and behaved more benignly to her.

Mrs Reiss then became very tearful and said that she knew what the 'real problem' was. It came as a complete surprise to the therapist when Mrs Reiss confessed that she was preoccupied with thoughts of her first husband and that she had never really overcome his death. She often visualized him in her imagination and said, 'I speak to him when I'm on my own.' Any mention of death or illness, especially cancer, caused her to think immediately of him.

Much time in the next few sessions was spent in discussing her first husband's death and Mrs Reiss' feelings about him. Ways in which she might act more assertively with her present husband were also explored.

Mrs Reiss improved again and became more assertive with her husband. She complained that he was still not keen on her going out. The psychologist spoke on the telephone to Mr Reiss on one occasion and he was clearly angry with his wife. He accused her of not practising because she had a 'lazy nature' and stated that she was not ill. When the psychologist mentioned that Mrs Reiss had expressed some concern about his health (he also had gall bladder stones) he replied, 'It's my business if I die.' The psychologist responded sympathetically to Mr Reiss and urged him to encourage Mrs Reiss to go out.

## Reassessment

Although Mrs Reiss' symptoms have fluctuated, she is now improving steadily. She has openly acknowledged feelings that she has kept private for years, presumably because her trust in those helping her has increased and she now feels more secure in treatment. It would be useful to reconsider her situation in order to see whether new lines of enquiry or treatment should be pursued.

## Diagnosis

In addition to the agoraphobia, obesity and hypertension it has become clear that Mrs Reiss has suffered from a long-standing, unresolved grief reaction following the death of her first husband. She has been unable to accept his death and has remained unusually preoccupied with his memory, which was immediately evoked by any reference to death.

## Aetiology

The problems that appeared to exist in Mr and Mrs Reiss' marriage have been confirmed by the contradictory reactions the psychologist observed when he spoke to Mr Reiss on the telephone. On one occasion he appeared sympathetic and expressed concern for his wife's illness and on another he blamed her completely for her problems. It is likely that Mr Reiss behaves in a way that tends to impede change in his wife. It would be short-sighted, however, to blame Mr Reiss' ambivalent attitude for the perpetuation of her symptoms. All marriages involve a complex pattern of interaction, since both partners contribute actively. Although this state may appear unsatisfactory to an outsider, it often represents a delicate balance. If it is disturbed the situation can deteriorate, or the partners may fear that it will. In Mrs Reiss' case it is plausible that her symptoms, by rooting her to her home, have made it impossible for her to abandon a relationship that she finds unsatisfactory. Her symptoms will have enabled her to maintain the security she managed to recreate for herself after the war. Mr Reiss may have been aware of her dissatisfaction and his fear of being abandoned by her would make his behaviour directed towards discouraging change more understandable.

It has also been revealed that Mr Reiss has a serious heart condition that appears to have caused him considerable worry. Given Mrs Reiss' preoccupation with her first husband, and her vulnerability to fear of death, this would have presumably been a considerable source of concern for her as well. It is surprising, in one so sensitive to illness, that she failed to mention her husband's heart condition about which he was obviously distressed. The reason for this omission is not clear, but may have been due to her understandable difficulty in facing the implication that he might die as well. Perhaps her unassertiveness with him was in part related to her fear that by resisting him she might hasten his demise.

Another factor that may have contributed to Mrs Reiss' illness is her daughter recently leaving her. Not only might this loss have been sad in itself, but it also meant that she was left alone with her husband.

### Further information

The significance of these, or other, aetiological and perpetuating factors should be explored by seeing the couple together, if this is possible.

### Management

The psychiatrist should provide Mrs Reiss with further opportunity to mourn her first husband's death by focusing on issues that evoke memories of him. It has also become increasingly clear that Mrs Reiss should be seen with her husband and more pressure should be brought to bear on them to attend together.

### Prognosis

Mrs Reiss should continue to improve, as she has already. However, the scope for improvement will depend upon the possibility of incorporating her husband in the treatment. It seems unlikely that she will ever completely come to terms with her losses, which have been so numerous and profound.

## Postscript

Her husband never attended the outpatient department. However, despite some minor setbacks, Mrs Reiss continued to make progress with her agoraphobic symptoms. She explored some of the ways in which she contributed to her husband's irritability with her. Thoughts about her first husband and her 'unforgiving nature' were identified as probably having an influence. Soon after, Mr Reiss expressed the desire to emigrate to Florida, which was contrary to her wishes. This had been a point of contention for some time, but not previously mentioned by the patient.

Although she responded to this more assertively than previously, the question remained unresolved at the end of treatment.

Mrs Reiss was discharged from the clinic after nine months, much improved. She was able to walk anywhere with minimal anxiety and could drive to any point in Manchester. She was still unable to approach escalators with total confidence, but felt that she could 'treat myself' for this. Her gains had been steady over the previous three months. Thoughts of her first husband were less frequent and she felt she had resolved much concerning his loss.

# Chapter 10

# I Have No Longer a Mind of My Own

## Mr Forrester

### Presenting complaint

Mrs Forrester telephoned the duty psychiatrist to ask for her husband to be seen urgently. She said that he had become increasingly depressed over the last few months and when he attended his last outpatient appointment two weeks previously, his psychiatrist prescribed fluoxetine. In spite of taking this regularly his mood had deteriorated and on the previous day he had made a noose of his tie, pulled it tight around his neck and then released it. On the day of the telephone call, while Mrs Forrester was visiting his mother, he broke a neighbour's window, cutting his wrist. On her return home she found a suicide note he had written to their ten-year-old son. The duty psychiatrist advised Mrs Forrester to bring him directly to the Accident and Emergency department. When they arrived, the following information was obtained from Mrs Forrester.

Mr Forrester had been a patient of the hospital for several years. Over the last few months his wife had become increasingly worried about him and had therefore brought forward his outpatient appointment. However, in spite of seeing his psychiatrist two weeks previously, when he was prescribed an antidepressant, his mood had deteriorated. He became increasingly taciturn and looked tense and miserable. He also began to talk more about how hopeless he felt about their marriage and began to sleep very badly. She had woken up on several occasions to find him sitting upright in bed during the early hours of the morning. At these times he stared bleakly out of the window. The previous week he woke up at 1.00 a.m. and said, 'Oh Christ, I can't think why you married me.' His appetite diminished considerably and he left at least half of his meal untouched. In contrast to his increasing withdrawal and apathy, Mr Forrester had begun to make more frequent sexual advances towards her over the last two weeks.

Mrs Forrester did not bring the suicide note with her. She could not remember exactly what it contained but it was written to their son and was basically an apology for feeling so hopeless.

The psychiatrist was unable to read Mr Forrester's records in detail before he examined him. However, he managed to obtain the following information from the summaries of Mr Forrester's previous admissions to hospital.

## Family history
His father was a general practitioner who died at the age of 59 from a coronary, when Mr Forrester was 12. He was said to have suffered from 'neurasthenia' and he spent the last year of his life in a nursing home. Although he was a rather distant man, he occasionally showed a very violent temper and shouted at his family. Mr Forrester's mother died at the age of 79, when Mr Forrester was 49. She was described as a kind, loving housewife who was very patient with the whole family. He had three siblings. Avril was eight years older than Mr Forrester, unmarried and died at the age of 36 from pneumonia. Alfred, who was six years older, was an airman who was shot down and went missing, presumed dead, at the end of the Second World War when Mr Forrester was 17. There was also an unmarried brother, Jack, two years older than Mr Forrester. He had been admitted for a few months to a nursing home when he was 48 with a 'nervous breakdown'. Apart from occasionally appearing a little 'odd', he had no further relapses and continued to lead a full and independent life.

## Personal history

Mr Forrester was born in Nottingham, where he spent a rather isolated childhood. He received private tuition until he was eight, when he started to attend the local boarding school. He never made any close friends, and immersed himself in his studies. He passed the entrance examination to Cambridge when he was 18 and read History. After he obtained his degree he taught history for a few years in a number of schools, but eventually decided to give this up. He then spent a few years travelling around South Africa before he returned to the United Kingdom, where he took a year's course in administration. For the past 15 years he had worked as a hospital archivist.

He met his wife, who was two years older, when he was 37. They married soon after meeting and their relationship was described as 'reasonably stable' until the last few years. They had one son, aged ten.

## Past medical history

At the age of four Mr Forrester fractured his leg in a car accident and this resulted in a permanent limp.

## Past psychiatric history

Mr Forrester had two brief spells of psychotherapy when he was aged 37 and 40. From the age of 42, he experienced fairly regular episodes of psychiatric illness, which required hospital inpatient treatment about every two years. On most of these admissions he was diagnosed as suffering from depression, but on one occasion a diagnosis of schizophrenia, and on two occasions a diagnosis of mania, had been made. Over the years he had received tricyclic antidepressants, haloperidol, electro-convulsive treatment and lithium carbonate. He had been maintained on lithium carbonate for the last two years and attended the outpatient department every few months in order to monitor both his mental state and his medication. Although his mood fluctuated during this time, most of the comments written about him by the doctors who saw him referred to his 'rather strange personality'.

## Previous personality

His wife described him as a withdrawn, shy, socially inept man who made few friends.

## Mental state examination

### Appearance and general behaviour

Mr Forrester was a tall, slightly stooped man with long, unkempt, white hair. His shirt collar was undone and he was not wearing a tie but he was otherwise dressed tidily. He sat with his head in his hands and looked tense and extremely dejected. His face had an agonized expression on it and he frequently grimaced. He spent the whole interview sitting still, looking at the floor.

### Speech

It was impossible to have a conversation with Mr Forrester. He answered most questions by shouting, 'I don't know.' When he spoke more fluently it was at a normal rate. He appeared to have formal thought disorder: when he was talking about his thoughts he said, 'I have no longer a mind of my own. I fear for the Queen's safety. I am not fit to be seen or heard.'

### Mood

Mr Forrester looked and sounded extremely miserable, but when he was asked if he was feeling depressed he shook his head vigorously. However, he broke down and sobbed after he described what was happening to his thoughts.

### Thought content

When he was asked how he felt he shouted, 'I don't know.' He shook his head when he was asked whether he felt angry or frightened. He was then asked whether he felt aggressive towards anyone and again shouted, 'Only with myself.' When the possibility of admission to hospital was suggested, he shouted out, 'No, no, no.'

*Abnormal beliefs and interpretations of events*

After the possibility of admission had been raised he went on to say, 'I don't know who my father is. I don't know what to think of him. I don't know whether he is a monster, too.' The psychiatrist then asked him whether he thought that he was a monster and he replied, 'Yes.' When he was asked what sort of a monster he said, 'God alone knows. He ought to, he made me.'

When he was asked about his thoughts Mr Forrester said, 'I think people can transfer their thoughts to my mind to make me do things I don't want to do, make me say things I don't want to say. I have no longer a mind of my own.'

*Abnormal experiences*

When he was talking about how he felt, Mr Forrester said, 'I feel as if I'm being pulled apart by some kind of a force.' He was then asked what this force was and replied, 'Ask my brother. I feel as if I'm being driven into the ground like a stake, but I don't know by whom.'

*Cognitive state*

This was not formally tested.

*Self-appraisal*

Mr Forrester was unable to discuss what was happening to him, but he made it clear that he did not want to be in hospital.

## Physical examination

This was not performed in the outpatient department, but it was noted that Mr Forrester's left arm was bandaged, apparently because of lacerations.

## Assessment

Mr Forrester's presentation is of a recent, severe alteration in mood and behaviour that has culminated in two episodes of self-harm, one of which was associated with him writing a suicide note. These changes have occurred in the context of a long-standing, cyclical illness, which has required fairly regular admission to hospital. The assessment therefore needs to address the severity of Mr Forrester's current state, the need for hospital admission and if necessary the possibility of invoking the Mental Health Act in order to obtain formal admission.

## Diagnosis

It is almost certain that Mr Forrester has developed an acute psychotic illness. His records show that he has had fairly regular episodes of psychotic illness over the last ten years. In addition, his wife describes deterioration in his mood and general behaviour over the last few months. She says that he has become increasingly withdrawn, has begun to express ideas of hopelessness and that his sleep and appetite have become seriously disturbed. These abnormalities have culminated in his suicide attempt. Finally, his mental state is extremely disturbed. He looks unhappy, is unable to give a coherent explanation for his recent behaviour, and what he does say suggests that he has experienced delusions and feels the victim of some kind of persecution. For example, when he describes himself as feeling 'pulled apart by some kind of force' and 'being driven into the ground like a stake'.

The nature of the psychotic illness is uncertain, because it has features consistent with both an affective disorder and a schizophrenic disorder. Both of these diagnoses have been made during previous episodes and the information obtained from the summaries is insufficient to resolve this uncertainty. However, it is his mood that appears to have been most affected by his illness, which suggests it is more likely to be an affective psychosis. This likelihood is reinforced by the description of recent changes in his sleep and eating and the fact that his illness appears to have had a fairly regular periodicity.

On the other hand, a diagnosis of schizophrenia has been made previously and persecutory ideas are prominent in this episode. An even more suspicious symptom is his description of thought insertion, which is said to be pathognomonic of a diagnosis of schizophrenia. However, this is not necessarily the case since Schneider's 'first rank symptoms' of schizophrenia can be found in cases of mania, particularly in the acute stages. Although Mr Forrester has shown no obvious manifestations of a manic illness during this episode, this diagnosis has been made in the past. Furthermore, his heightened sexual activity, which contrasts with his general sense of retardation, raises the possibility that he has a mixture of depressive and manic symptoms (a mixed affective state) that often occurs in acute affective illnesses.

## Aetiology

Mr Forrester appears to have a familial predisposition to psychiatric illness. His father suffered from what the family describes as 'neurasthenia' (weakness of the nerves) that may have led to him spending the last years of his life in a nursing home. His brother has also had a 'nervous breakdown', which required treatment in a psychiatric hospital. In addition to the possibility that Mr Forrester might have inherited a predisposition to psychiatric illness, it may be that exposure to his father's unpredictable and volatile mood also influenced his personality development. His wife described Mr Forrester as generally an isolated and depressive person. Although she did not meet him before he suffered his first psychiatric episode, this tendency towards isolation appears to extend back into his early childhood. This raises the possibility that Mr Forrester has a schizoid personality, which would colour any psychiatric illness he might develop. Epidemiological studies suggest that lack of sociability during childhood increases the risk of subsequent psychotic illness in adulthood.

No obvious precipitants of this episode have been identified. His illness has previously shown a periodicity of approximately two years, which is additional support for some underlying biological vulnerability. There is also the possibility that Mr Forrester has not been taking his medication as prescribed and that this might have contributed to his relapse.

## Further information

In order to clarify the diagnosis it is necessary to define more clearly Mr Forrester's current mental state. It is also important to obtain more details of his mental state during previous admissions. This should show the extent to which his abnormal beliefs and behaviour are consistent with an affective or a schizophrenic illness.

A full physical examination needs to be performed, particularly in view of his efforts at self-harm.

It might also prove useful to find out more about the details of both his brother's and his father's psychiatric episodes. If they also showed features of a psychotic disorder this would increase the likelihood of a constitutional vulnerability.

More information is also required about his personal and developmental history. In particular, his reasons for changing his job and the quality of degree he obtained would provide a clearer picture of his personality and his capabilities before his first episode of psychiatric illness.

Further detail is also needed about the events in Mr Forrester's life during the time leading up to this episode. Given Mrs Forrester's comments about his personality it would not be surprising to find that their marriage had been under considerable strain. It may also be relevant that his first serious psychiatric episode occurred at the time his son was born.

Blood levels of lithium will need to be obtained. These may show the extent to which Mr Forrester has been cooperating with his medical treatment.

*Management*

There are important clinical indications for admitting Mr Forrester immediately. First, he is suffering from a serious exacerbation of a psychiatric illness that warrants urgent treatment. Second, treatment as an outpatient has already failed to prevent a considerable deterioration. Third, there is evidence to suggest that he is a danger to himself. Within the last 24 hours there have been two episodes of self-harm and he has written a suicide note to his son. These factors suggest that he should be admitted to hospital urgently and that when this takes place he will have to be closely observed. Finally, he neither thinks he is ill nor believes he needs psychiatric treatment. Since he is not only seriously ill, but also a considerable danger to himself as a result of this, Mr Forrester should be admitted to a ward where special attention can be paid to his nursing care. In view of the presumptive diagnosis his antidepressant medication should also be continued as response is often only seen after two to three weeks of treatment, lithium blood levels need to be obtained and an antipsychotic should be added to his medication in view of his symptoms. Mr Forrester's reaction to admission suggests that this might require formal procedures under the Mental Health Act if all attempts to gain his cooperation fail.

*Prognosis*

Although Mr Forrester is seriously ill, it seems likely that he will recover from this episode as he has done previously. What is uncertain is how long this recovery will take, how complete it will be and how vulnerable Mr Forrester will remain to further relapses. A clearer picture should emerge once more information has become available.

## Further details

When the duty psychiatrist made clear his intention to admit Mr Forrester urgently he agreed to come into hospital voluntarily. Following admission, it was possible to examine his psychiatric records in more detail and to obtain further information from him and from his wife. Olanzapine, 10mg daily, was added to his medication.

Mr Forrester's early recollections were fairly happy ones. However, he had no memory of playing with his siblings nor of having any close friends. It became clearer that his father's psychiatric illness had been incapacitating and it caused him to spend the last year of his life in a nursing home. However, no further details about this or his brother's illness were obtained.

Mr Forrester had always immersed himself in his studies to the exclusion of any social life. This continued at Cambridge, where he obtained a second-class Classics degree. When he left Cambridge, he applied for war service but was rejected because of his limp. He then taught for several years. Although he initially found this quite enjoyable, he had considerable difficulty maintaining discipline and it was for this reason that he gave it up. He then decided to take up a course in administration and when he completed this he travelled to South Africa. He said that this was because he felt unsettled in England and when he left he had intended to settle in South Africa permanently. He found life there more relaxed and he was able to make several friends, but in spite of this he found himself missing England increasingly and therefore returned after seven years. He remained unemployed for two years after his return and then obtained his current work.

He generally enjoyed his work, although he occasionally felt that he was 'stuck in a rut'. His employers described him as having been a 'painstaking and conscientious worker' and said that they never found any cause for concern about him until the time of his first 'breakdown', when they noticed an increasing number of errors in his work. At that time they also noticed him becoming quite withdrawn and on occasions either falling asleep or just wandering away from work. After his first admission to hospital he returned to work, although there were several periods of sick leave during subsequent relapses. His employers were very sympathetic to his difficulties and kept his job open for him. However, he was transferred to another department for what were described as 'administrative reasons'. One advantage of his current job was that it provided Mr Forrester with a considerable amount of spare time to pursue his hobbies of writing short plays and poetry.

Before he met his wife he had several girlfriends, but none of these relationships were serious or intimate. His wife said that when she first met him she 'felt sorry for him', but also went on to say that she did not realize 'how difficult he could be' until after they married. She was particularly bothered by his tendency to withdraw from any active involvement in the family. Although they never had a frequent sexual relationship, this had become totally non-existent over the previous three years. Both Mr and Mrs Forrester said that this was no cause for concern. When they married they did not plan to have any children but Mr Forrester said that although he was not closely involved in his son's upbringing, he 'accepted' and 'felt responsible' for him.

In addition to writing, his interests were intellectual and unusual. He had always been fascinated by languages and once began to learn Esperanto, out of which he developed ideas to create a language of his own. At the time of his first psychiatric breakdown he became interested in a religious cult that was attempting to reconcile all religions under one banner.

## Past psychiatric history

Mr Forrester's first admission to a psychiatric hospital took place when he was 42. He was diagnosed as suffering from endogenous depression and was reported to have responded well to electro-convulsive treatment. A few months later, he was readmitted to another psychiatric hospital, where a diagnosis of schizophrenia was made, based upon the presence of 'bizarre, delusional ideas'. However, it was noted at that time that these occurred in the context of a depressive mood. The diagnosis was subsequently changed to one of endogenous depression and he was given a further course of electro-convulsive therapy in addition to trifluoperazine and dothiepin. One year later, he was readmitted with a diagnosis of depression, which again responded to a course of electro-convulsive therapy. Two years later, he took an overdose of antidepressants and was readmitted to hospital.

Following this overdose he suffered a grand mal seizure. He later developed an elated mood with considerable overactivity, as a result of which a diagnosis of mania was made. At this time he was treated with haloperidol and he appeared to remain well for a further two years. He was then readmitted compulsorily for a three-day period of assessment, which was extended to a one-year treatment order on account of his continuing unpredictable behaviour. There were frequent comments in the notes about his becoming embroiled in arguments with staff over whether he needed to be in hospital and receive treatment. He was reported to have left the ward without warning on several occasions and the nursing staff found him very uncooperative. There were frequent comments in their records about their difficulty in getting to know him. The final diagnosis on this admission was mania.

Since his last admission Mr Forrester had often failed to keep his outpatient appointments and frequently wrote letters to the doctors who looked after him. These discussed, amongst other things, the value (or lack of it) that he placed upon his contact with the hospital, the psychological basis of illness and other philosophical issues. His letter writing appeared to alter during his 'manic' phase. The letters became not only more frequent and longer, but more rambling with some flight of ideas. For example, one letter described a profound religious experience, then personal and sexual experiences, then problems with medication, then a review of important biographical dates in his life, and then a train journey. This was closely written on five sides of paper in two colours of ink.

Further enquiry about the events leading up to Mr Forrester's recent deterioration revealed that he had started a course on administration six months beforehand. However, he felt unable to continue after two days and gave it up. Mrs Forrester believed that his mood began to deteriorate at about this time. No other specific stresses were revealed.

The various doctors who saw Mr Forrester and his wife in the outpatient department commented on Mrs Forrester's anxiety about her husband, in particular the fact that she frequently telephoned the hospital to voice her worries about him. There were also comments about how his mood had fluctuated during the previous two years. However, most of their notes referred to his 'rather strange, withdrawn personality'.

## Physical examination

A complete physical examination revealed evidence of weight loss, a superficial three-inch laceration of his left arm, and a fixed flexion deformity of his right knee, but no other abnormality.

## Special investigations

Mr Forrester's serum lithium level was 0.5 micromol/l. Although this was just within the therapeutic range for the laboratory (0.5–1.5 micromol/l) it was lower than the level Mr Forrester had maintained during the previous four years (0.6–0.8 micromol/l).

Otherwise all investigations were normal.

## Mental state examination

*Appearance and general behaviour*

Following his admission Mr Forrester took very little care of his appearance, and remained unkempt and unshaven. He ate poorly, which he attributed to an aversion to meat. He was reported to be sleeping restlessly. He developed no rapport with anyone on the ward and when interviewed he either paced restlessly around or sat upright, unblinking in a chair, staring at the floor with his legs crossed and hands clasped tensely.

*Speech*

During the first week, he offered no spontaneous conversation and always gave terse answers to questions. However, he became a little more forthcoming towards the end of his second week in hospital.

*Mood*

During the first week of his admission he consistently conveyed to the ward staff a sense of desolation and hopelessness. He said that he felt as if he were in 'cold storage' and that admission to hospital had been 'an ordeal I have to experience', and although 'it could conceivably have a useful purpose in the long run', he saw his 'previous life as having been a preparation for this'. He thought that he deserved to have this experience and saw it as a punishment for having been rude to his father, as well as for having blasphemed when he was admitted to hospital four years previously. He made numerous allusions to suicide, saying that life was not worth living and that he would 'welcome the opportunity for suicide' because he would be 'better off out of the way'. One way of achieving this would be to 'sacrifice myself as a hero rather than being a coward' and he was therefore prepared to offer himself for 'euthanasia'.

*Thought content*

He expressed an interest in symbolism, which he thought conveyed messages. He gave as an example, 'a frog, which is ignorant of the underworld'. When asked to explain what this meant, he replied, 'It has something to do with croaking. If you croak you are finished.' He then said that someone at a religious festival he had attended a few weeks previously, who wore some clothes with a picture of a frog on the back, reminded him of this.

*Abnormal beliefs and interpretations of events*

Mr Forrester seemed very suspicious and expressed the belief that he was being 'organized by someone else, possibly for historical purposes'. There seemed to him to be 'a purpose behind what was going on', although he did not know what this was and thought that 'only God could provide an answer'. He wondered if God had made use of the Devil to test him. A week after his admission, he said that at the time of his admission he 'felt framed' and 'imagined' that his room had been bugged. At that time he said that someone was listening because 'I gave a transmission, a couple of sonnets and a short poem in Russian. I wasn't going to give away any secrets – I can't remember what they were. It always comes back to loyalty.' He also said that he imagined he was the 'pretender to the throne'. In addition to these thoughts, he felt that everything had a double meaning 'like being in a film', but he was unable to elaborate further on this. When efforts were made to establish how firmly he held these ideas, he always deflected this line of enquiry by saying that he used to believe these things or that they were imaginary.

*Abnormal experiences*

None were elicited. He did not refer again to his previous experience of thought insertion.

*Cognitive state*

This was never formally tested, apart from confirming that Mr Forrester was orientated in time and space.

*Self-appraisal*

Soon after his admission Mr Forrester said, 'I don't honestly feel unwell.' Ten days later, he said, 'I was certainly ill one week ago, but I am sane now.'

## Nursing observations

All the nursing staff commented on his rather cold, empty and distant personality that made it difficult for them to empathize with his situation.

## Reassessment

Although not all the questions raised in the initial formulation have been answered, a consistent view of Mr Forrester, extending back over nearly ten years, has emerged.

*Diagnosis*

There is now little doubt that Mr Forrester is suffering from a bipolar affective disorder, current episode depression with psychotic features (ICD10); or bipolar II disorder (DSMIV). He conveys an intensity of hopelessness about himself and his future and the many delusions he describes all have a distinctive depressive colouring and appear to have arisen out of this mood change, rather than being the cause of it. These delusions are quite persecutory, since he believes he is at the centre of some religious conspiracy and that he is being 'organized' by some outside agent. In addition they have a grandiose quality because Mr Forrester believes he has been singled out and is going to be a part of history.

This grandiose quality raises the suspicion that there is a manic element to Mr Forrester's current illness. This is reinforced by another symptom suggestive of mania that has been noted. Mr Forrester makes an association between a frog, the underworld and death in a characteristic 'flight of ideas' linked by, amongst other things, the pun on the word 'croaked'. This admixture of manic and depressive symptoms, in the context of a chronic episodic illness with both depressive and manic swings, defines this as a mixed episode (DSMIV).

It seems that Mr Forrester may have experienced 'thought broadcasting' early on during his admission. Although this is one of the 'first rank symptoms' of schizophrenia, as previously discussed, such symptoms can occur during a manic illness. This explanation is further supported by the previous descriptions of 'bizarre thoughts' that occurred in earlier episodes, which have nevertheless followed the pattern of a cyclical affective illness.

The additional information that has been obtained also suggests that Mr Forrester has a schizoid personality. He appears to have had a life-long tendency to social withdrawal and isolation and has never had any intense emotional involvement with another person, including his wife and son. In particular he described his relationship with his son in terms of responsibility, rather than concern. Furthermore, he has always shown interest in rather abstruse matters, such as developing a new language or the philosophical aspects of religion. Although these features are not in themselves necessarily manifestations of a psychiatric disturbance, when they play such a prominent part in an individual's character they suggest considerable eccentricity. These schizoid attributes seem to have coloured Mr Forrester's psychotic episodes when they have occurred, giving them what has been referred to as their 'bizarre' or 'schizophrenic' qualities.

## Aetiology

Establishing the severity of his father's illness reinforces the relevance of a familial factor in Mr Forrester's illness. He may also have inherited a schizoid tendency from his father that could well have been reinforced by his rather isolated upbringing.

Mr Forrester's recent deterioration appears to have been associated with his starting a course that he failed to complete. From his wife's account, it is possible that this setback may have triggered off this episode, although it could also have been an early symptom of it.

There is also the likelihood that Mr and Mrs Forrester's marriage is under considerable stress as a result of his personality and his vulnerability to illness. She has made several criticisms about his lack of involvement and has expressed disappointment at the way their marriage has turned out. Although no specific details have been revealed, it is also possible that Mrs Forrester has been putting her husband under increasing pressure on account of this. Given his personality he would find it very difficult to cope with intense emotional demands and this might have also been a factor contributing to his deterioration.

His previous records contain no mention of any specific environmental triggers. However, his first psychotic episode did occur within the first year of his son's birth and it is possible that the additional emotional demands of a small child might have contributed to this episode, too.

Finally, the blood tests have shown that his medication is at the lower therapeutic level. Given the stresses discussed above and his apparent cyclical vulnerability, this relative lack of medication may also have contributed to his relapse.

## Further information

It will be important to obtain a much more detailed account of Mr and Mrs Forrester's relationship. This should include an estimation of its strengths as well as its weaknesses. It is unclear how much support Mrs Forrester is giving her husband and whether she may be making unrealistic demands of him, given his personality and psychological vulnerability.

More details should be obtained about the course that appears to have been associated with Mr Forrester's deterioration. In particular, it should be clarified whether this did in fact precede his relapse.

## Management

Mr Forrester will need to remain in a ward where he can be given high intensity nursing care until he is no longer a danger to himself and shows a capacity to cooperate with treatment. It would probably be wise to keep him there until it is clear that he is not developing a full-blown manic episode, particularly in the light of his previous difficulty in cooperating with treatment. Should he seem to be developing a manic state, his fluoxetine will need to be discontinued, as this has been linked to exacerbations of mania in a few patients with propensity to bipolar affective disorder.

The possibility of electro-convulsive treatment should be considered, since it has been shown to be useful for Mr Forrester in the past. However, he has already shown signs of improvement during his first two weeks in hospital, when he was known to be receiving adequate doses of fluoxetine, lithium carbonate and olanzapine. Although a case can be put forward for giving electro-convulsive treatment as well, there seems little point in doing this while he continues to improve. He will need to continue with fluoxetine for at least six months after he has recovered from this episode and to continue with his lithium carbonate indefinitely, with appropriate blood level monitoring, because he has shown vulnerability to regular, serious relapses. The dose of olanzapine could be gradually reduced over the first three months.

Mr Forrester should be encouraged to return to work following recovery. Assuming that his employers are prepared to keep his job available for him, his work environment seems particularly suitable for someone of his personality and vulnerability in that it appears to be emotionally undemanding.

Further treatment of the couple will probably need to be educational, helping them to avoid situations that might precipitate further breakdown. The need for this has already been demonstrated by the frequency with which Mrs Forrester telephones the hospital to communicate her anxiety about her husband. It may be that more fundamental interpersonal issues will become aired, but this could have disastrous consequences given Mr Forrester's personality and it may be better to avoid too deep an exploration.

It may be necessary to advise Mr Forrester to avoid certain situations to which he is vulnerable. An example of this might turn out to be courses like the one that was associated with his current deterioration.

*Prognosis*

It is likely that Mr Forrester will recover from this episode after a few months in hospital as he has done on previous occasions. However, there is a considerable risk that he will swing into a manic phase once his depression lifts. If this follows the previous pattern, then it will be associated with considerable conflict between Mr Forrester and the ward staff. In the longer term Mr Forrester appears to be vulnerable to a relapse at intervals of approximately two years. The possibility of preventing this will depend upon very closely monitoring his mental state, potential social triggers and medication.

Given his employer's previous cooperation and the lack of stress placed upon him at work, it is likely that Mr Forrester will be able to return there.

There is a clear danger that Mr and Mrs Forrester's marriage will break down, partly on account of his illness and partly because of his personality difficulties. The likelihood of this happening cannot be ascertained until more information has been obtained about the couple's relationship.

## Postscript

Mr Forrester remained in hospital for five months and his recovery was stormy. He had marked mood swings, which might have been partly attributable to a muddle over his medication. He embarked upon a relationship with a female patient, which caused his wife considerable distress. However, his mental state was controlled with a mixture of lithium carbonate, fluoxetine and olanzapine. In spite of improvement, he remained an extremely impenetrable individual, who continued to be preoccupied with philosophical conundrums.

Efforts were made to embark upon conjoint assessment and counselling, but these were not maintained. Mrs Forrester had considerable difficulty in attending, which was heightened by her husband's flirtation on the ward. Eventually Mr Forrester went on a fortnight's holiday with his wife and returned to his home and to work without reporting back to the ward.

Six years later Mr Forrester had not required readmission. He suffered several relapses associated, as before, with an alteration in his letter writing, but these were controlled by an increase in his medication. He managed to cope with the stresses imposed by his mother-in-law's death and his retirement. According to his employers, he continued to function well until his retirement, when he was offered part-time, unpaid employment.

On two occasions, Mrs Forrester 'offered' to leave her husband because she believed that she 'contributed to his illness'. However, over several years their relationship appeared to settle down considerably.

Mr Forrester's brother wrote to his psychiatrist after his discharge suggesting that 'a mixture of drug intoxication and vitamin imbalance' could explain his problem. He thought this could also have contributed to his own, and their father's, illness. This letter was as disjointed and obscure as were Mr Forrester's during his manic phases.

# Chapter 11

# My House is Bugged

## Mr Butler

### Presenting complaint

Mr Butler's general practitioner referred him to a psychiatric emergency clinic because he was 'going through another episode of suicidal thoughts'. The GP's letter stated, 'For about five years he has suffered from profound mental disturbance, with withdrawal, depersonalization, depression and paranoia.' A confident diagnosis of paranoid schizophrenia was made in the emergency clinic, the risk of suicide was noted, and Mr Butler was referred to see a consultant in the outpatient department. The consultant thought that the correct diagnosis was depressive illness in a sensitive personality and made arrangements for admission.

Mr Butler himself had the following complaints: 'my house is being bugged', 'electronic noises are being made', and 'wind effects are occurring outside my house when there was no wind'. He also said that he had been frightened when 'something happened in my head like a shock wave'. The police were somehow mixed up with it, he thought. The history, obtained during the course of a two-month admission, was as follows.

Mr Butler had been becoming hard of hearing for about ten years. Five years before admission he became preoccupied with the idea that people were staring at him and that the police were following him. His beer drinking increased and, later that year, the police arrested him for being drunk and disorderly. This convinced him that his suspicions of the police were correct.

Four years before admission Mr Butler took an overdose of a prescribed hypnotic whilst feeling 'depressed', and was admitted to a psychiatric hospital for the first time. He did not return to his job and was re-admitted after three months. He had then worked only intermittently, in a succession of jobs, each shorter than the last. The police arrested him again on a drunk and disorderly charge, and shortly after this, 18 months before the present admission, his feeling that the police were everywhere, 'putting pressure' on him, had become so intense that he felt that he could not work.

Eight months before admission he cut his wrist with a razor blade and then made preparations to hang himself, although eventually decided against doing so. He was again admitted to a psychiatric hospital, via a casualty department, but discharged himself after three days.

Since that time he had not worked but occupied himself at home reading magazines and doing crossword puzzles. He described himself as feeling 'continuously worried and depressed'.

## Family history

Mr Butler's father, aged 63, had recently retired on medical grounds from the post office where he was a sorting office supervisor, but continued working as a part-time clerk in a builder's yard. He suffered from hypertension and angina. Mr Butler described him as a self-contained, rather quiet man. He was in the habit of going to the pub twice a week with his son, and they shared an interest in football. Mr Butler's mother was also 63. She seemed a more outgoing woman who was the boss of the family and 'doted' on Mr Butler. She had continued to work part time as a school dinner-lady after she passed the age of retirement. Mr Butler had two siblings. (The first-born child, a brother, had died at birth.) An older brother, married with six children, had emigrated to Australia, where he was working as a storeman. An older sister was married to a local electrician and had one child.

Mr Butler described his upbringing as having been 'warm and happy'. There was no family history of psychiatric disorder but a cousin had epilepsy and was described as 'violent'.

## Personal history

Mr Butler had lived throughout his life in a market town in the north of England. He was born in hospital by Caesarean section after a trial of labour had failed because of pelvic disproportion. There were no other perinatal complications. He was an unusually shy and timid child who became anxious easily. He disliked being alone but otherwise his development was normal; he enjoyed the company of other children and particularly liked sports. After some initial apprehension he enjoyed school and was always a model pupil. He got on with everyone, both teachers and pupils, and became a prefect at secondary school. His academic record was good and he passed three GCSEs at the age of 16, in history, art and technical drawing. He wanted to stay on at school but his mother insisted that he went out to work, to supplement the family income.

After leaving school when he was 16 Mr Butler joined a brewery and worked in the stocktaking department for 12 years. His work entailed travelling and making a complete on-the-spot inventory of the firm's stock and estimating its value. His ability to perform rapid calculations, his reliability and, especially, his probity were much thought of and he was promoted to a position of seniority, shortly before his first breakdown.

There was an occasion, when Mr Butler was 11, when he had engaged in mutual masturbation with another boy at school. He experienced his first ejaculation when he was 14. He was, however, very shy with girls and despite occasional 'dates' did not so much as kiss a girl until he was 20. When he was 16 Mr Butler became infatuated with a young woman who lived locally and he would stand outside her house to try and catch glimpses of her undressing. On several occasions he stood deliberately close behind her at the bus stop and rubbed his body against hers. For a few years after this he would rub himself against, or touch knees with, women who attracted him when he was travelling on crowded trains. This activity did not outlast his adolescence and it never led to police attention. He exhibited himself, on one occasion, after drinking heavily in his early 20s.

Mr Butler had one experience of sexual intercourse, with his only girl-friend, at the age of 22. They split up shortly after. At the time of admission his only sexual outlet was masturbation. He masturbated two to three times a week, usually whilst looking at 'girlie' magazines. He kept a collection of these, and felt humiliated when, shortly before admission, his father discovered them.

Like his father, Mr Butler had been a regular beer-drinker since adolescence. His occupation facilitated his drinking but it was only towards the end of his work for the brewery that he began to drink heavily every day, both at lunchtime and in the evening. For some time before his admission he did not have enough money to drink every day, but developed the habit of drinking at least five pints of beer every Saturday and Sunday.

## Life situation

Mr Butler and his parents had lived throughout his life in a three-bedroom council home. He contributed some rent, but did very little at home, relying on his mother to clean his room, and to do his cooking and washing.

## Past medical history

He was found to be deaf more than ten years before.

## Past psychiatric history

Mr Butler first saw a psychiatrist at the age of 28 when he was admitted as a day patient following medical treatment for an overdose of barbiturate. He attended hospital daily for three weeks and a diagnosis of 'acute paranoid reaction in a sensitive schizoid personality' was made. He was given no medication. Alcohol was thought to be a precipitant and he was advised to reduce his drinking. He was referred to an outpatient therapy group.

Informal inpatient admission, for investigations, was arranged four months later and he was in hospital for three weeks. Mr Butler was given no medication and the notes stated that there was 'no overt evidence of paranoid psychosis manifested on the ward' and 'no evidence of alcoholism'. Outpatient follow-up was recommended, but he did not attend.

The third admission followed medical treatment for self-inflicted wrist lacerations, as already described. Mr Butler discharged himself after five days during which he received no drug treatment. The diagnosis of 'reactive depression related to feelings of sexual inadequacy' was made.

## Previous personality

His mother described him as having always been 'very shy and sensitive. An introvert.' However, he was held in high esteem at work and school, and 'never lost a day's work'. She remarked also on his obedience, his many male friends, and his lack of girlfriends. Mr Butler preferred to stay at home when he could and once described himself as 'a bird who can't leave the nest'.

## Mental state examination

### Appearance and general behaviour

Mr Butler was a short man of athletic build. His clothes were clean and his hair short and neatly combed. He sat in a tense posture and moved his body very little, although he smiled a lot. His voice was soft, and rather slow. He was rather passive during the interview, but ready to do anything that was asked of him.

### Speech

His speech was normal, if slightly monosyllabic.

### Mood

Mr Butler seemed slightly tense but was not overtly agitated. He described himself as 'a bit on the low side'. His appetite was normal and his weight steady. He had difficulty in falling asleep and his ruminations (to be described below) were worse at night. He woke later rather than earlier, and he had no diurnal variation of mood. His suicidal preoccupations had disappeared after admission.

## Thought content

Mr Butler's conversation constantly reverted to the police and thought that they were watching and following him. In situations where he felt less guarded Mr Butler would explain that the police were interested in his sexual activities, either because they knew of his previous frotteurism, or because he was considered to be homosexual, or sometimes because 'they think I will assault a child'. These thoughts were so persistent that they interfered with Mr Butler's attention.

## Abnormal beliefs and interpretations of events

Mr Butler imbued many aspects of his environment with abnormal significance, feeling it to be filled with personal references to himself. When he saw a child he thought that the police had arranged for the child to be there as a test of his sexuality. He also thought that the television and the newspapers made disguised reference to his predicament, for example by broadcasting songs in which the word 'baby' was used.

Mr Butler believed that he could tell that his case was well known to an individual person by the way that person looked at him, or by the way that fellow patients held their trays at dinner, or by gestures that they made with their hands. Casual conversations that he overheard took on a special meaning for him, and such a conversation had precipitated his recent overdose.

He was convinced that his parents' flat was bugged, and that television cameras controlled by the police were observing him.

Mr Butler had recently imagined having sex with children, but believed that the police had put these thoughts into his mind. He had also occasionally linked the exacerbation of his ruminations at night with the upstairs neighbour turning off the lights, and on one occasion said, 'This man could turn the switch on me.'

*Abnormal experiences*

One of Mr Butler's complaints, as already mentioned, was of visual 'wind effects' in the absence of wind. These only lasted a day and were closely associated with hearing noises in his ears like 'wind or electronic noise'. These noises never sounded like words but were usually described as 'ringing' and felt by Mr Butler to originate in his ears.

*Cognitive state*

Mr Butler's orientation, attention and recall were normal. His retention of a short address was poor. He performed serial subtraction accurately and unusually quickly, and seemed of above average intelligence.

*Self-appraisal*

Mr Butler was curiously ambivalent about the nature of his condition. Whilst being convinced that his suspicions of the police were well founded, at the same time he would say that they were too fantastic to be true and that he had 'a complex'.

## Physical examination

The only abnormalities detected were short sight fully corrected by spectacles and bilateral deafness, worse on the left. Sound was conducted better through bone than air in both ears.

## Assessment

Mr Butler is a 34-year-old single, unemployed man who lives with his parents in a small council flat. He has a ten-year history of increasing deafness, and a five-year history of fluctuating ideas of reference and persecutory beliefs, especially involving the police. He has made two recent attempts on his life and is a heavy drinker. As a result of his disturbance he has had multiple admissions that have resulted in a variety of diagnoses but have not led to effective treatment. The first priority is to clarify the diagnosis and this will entail accurately defining the signs and symptoms he presents.

## Diagnosis

Mr Butler has delusions of reference. He is also probably hallucinating: he has described inexplicable visual experiences (seeing plants moving outside the window when there was no wind) and hearing 'electronic noises'. The noises, which he locates in his ear, may be related to his deafness, and be due to his hearing difficulty. However, tinnitus is unlikely to occur in conductive deafness. A further possibility is that these are auditory hallucinations.

The prominence of delusions in Mr Butler's illness, coupled with the absence of other disabling signs and symptoms of psychosis, justify the descriptive term paranoid state or paranoid psychosis. (Both usages of the term – the original one of 'delusional', and the more modern one of relating to ideas of persecution – are applicable to Mr Butler.) Paranoid states may occur alone or in combination with the signs and symptoms of some organic psychoses, depression or of schizophrenia.

There is no evidence that Mr Butler has ever suffered from epilepsy, or that he has ever abused drugs (two common causes of an organic paranoid state), nor is there any sign of cognitive impairment. There is therefore no support for the diagnosis of organic psychosis.

Although it is uncommon for a depressive psychosis to take this form, it does sometimes happen in patients with sensitive or suspicious pre-morbid personality traits. Where the pre-morbid personality is markedly abnormal even quite mild depression may produce a paranoid state. This is consistent with Mr Butler's complaint of feeling depressed and his ruminations about previous minor sexual transgressions. However, Mr Butler's suicide attempts are not diagnostically specific, since despair about the future may also occur in sufferers from other serious psychiatric disorders, such as schizophrenia. There is also no significant evidence of primary depression, such as weight loss, diurnal variation of mood, or sleep disturbance. He did not feel he was to blame about his previous sexual behaviour, but the object of unfair discrimination by the police on account of it.

Persecutory beliefs, which arise in sensitive individuals like Mr Butler who become depressed, usually disappear when the depression lifts. Mr Butler's mood, however, appears to have lightened after hospital admission but without a corresponding change in his delusions. A depressive disorder is not therefore the most likely cause of his symptoms.

Mr Butler's symptoms are all consistent with schizophrenia and the paranoid sub-type would be applicable in his case. However, there is no definite evidence of this disorder, even though some of Mr Butler's delusions, such as his conviction that patients know about his previous sex offences, are 'primary', in that they were not prompted by abnormal experiences. It is not clear whether his first delusion, that the police were following him, was based on a misperception or whether it was a delusional inference from a normal perception. The latter, a 'delusional perception', is characteristic of schizophrenia, whereas the former is not.

On one occasion Mr Butler said, 'The police put these thoughts [sexual thoughts towards children] in my head.' The examining psychiatrist thought this was an example of thought insertion. Since it is one of Schneider's first-rank symptoms its presence would reinforce the diagnosis of schizophrenia. However, without knowing how the thoughts were put into Mr Butler's head, it is possible that he simply meant that some things that the police did suggested these thoughts to him.

A paranoid state characterized by delusions but not hallucinations, a delusional disorder or 'paranoia', may sometimes result from the insidious elaboration of normal preoccupations until these dominate an individual's thinking and give rise to delusional beliefs about, and misinterpretations of, their experience. The development of Mr Butler's suspicions about the police has this character. They developed in the context of his exaggerated guilty ruminations about past sexual deviations, and were exacerbated by his arrest on a charge of being drunk and disorderly. Chance sightings of policemen were subsequently explained by this belief: they were on the look-out for him, and knew his movements because they had installed bugging devices in his flat. The police's interest in him was also used to explain difficulties in relationships with workmates who were 'in the know'.

However, the seeds of paranoia are often plausible, because they grow in areas that are particularly open to doubt such as religion, physical health, or justice. Mr Butler gives several instances of new extensions of a delusional system that arrived as sudden convictions without any proper evidence; for example, the way a fellow patient held a tray showed that he was 'in the know'. This would be an unusual feature of paranoia.

Apart from possible thought insertion, there are no definite, pathognomonic features of schizophrenia and this diagnosis is therefore tentative. This is a fairly common situation since many features, such as thought disorder and social deterioration, are less marked in the paranoid than the other sub-types of schizophrenia.

### Aetiology

Although this can only be determined when a definite diagnosis has been made there are some factors that seem of likely importance.

Mr Butler has been a heavy weekend beer drinker for a number of years, and increased his consumption as his illness deteriorated. However, this seems to have been in response to his symptoms rather than a cause of them and there is no evidence that he was physically dependent on alcohol. Nevertheless, regular heavy drinking is known to contribute to the development of paranoid states.

Mr Butler was timid and prone to anxiety as a child, and in adolescence he was abnormally shy and unassertive. These are some of the features of a schizoid personality, which predisposes to the development of schizophrenia. His lack of social experience, limited social contact and sexual naivety is likely to have facilitated the development of his eccentric ideas and increased his anxiety in social encounters. Mr Butler's deafness may also have increased his social anxiety and provided opportunities for misinterpretation of other people's remarks.

There is no family history of schizophrenia and the abuse of drugs can also be ruled out of the possible causes. However, Mr Butler did have a complicated birth, and perinatal trauma is probably a vulnerability factor.

The factors considered might all have contributed to Mr Butler first becoming ill, although none account for the timing of its onset. All the likely precipitants are psychological, including the stress of changing his job to one requiring more responsibility.

A more important consideration, relevant to practical management, is what causes Mr Butler's relapses. Current stresses at home, drinking difficulties at work and concern about sexuality should all be considered. The history obtained so far is not sufficiently clear for any of these factors to be singled out.

The content of Mr Butler's delusions is strongly influenced by his concern about his sexuality. However, it cannot yet be concluded that conflict about his sexual feelings is an especially important source of stress.

### Further information

Mr Butler's deafness needs assessment with a view to treatment. In practice it is probably best that he is referred to an ENT specialist.

Several areas of the history need further investigation. Knowledge of Mr Butler's development and pre-morbid activities and interests is somewhat sketchy, and a confident diagnosis about his pre-morbid personality cannot be made. Nor is the history of his illness sufficiently well documented for the aetiologically important factors to be identified. It would also be useful to interview Mr Butler with his family to observe how they interact and ascertain whether stress at home may have contributed to his illness.

Some features of Mr Butler's mental state, particularly the nature of his abnormal experiences, need clarification. For example, does he experience auditory hallucinations?

Another important investigation is to observe Mr Butler's response to treatment, including hospital admission. The effects of living away from home, of increased social contact, of reducing alcohol consumption, and of improved auditory acuity (assuming that it is treatable) also need to be tested.

Blood should be sent as a routine for syphilis serology, and urine for a drug screen. Routine physical examinations should be carried out to exclude the possibility of concurrent physical illness.

### Management

Mr Butler's management will depend on a more precise determination of diagnosis and aetiology.

In the short term a decision has already been made to admit him partly because of his suicidal preoccupations. Although these have disappeared since admission it is wise not to forget them until Mr Butler has been effectively treated. Medical and nursing staff should therefore be particularly alert to any deterioration in Mr Butler's mood. Medication may be started once a definite view has been formed about diagnosis. It is also important that he does not become more disabled as a result of inactivity on the ward. An occupational therapy programme may help to prevent this, especially if it can be made relevant to his work.

Making available other social roles, such as patient representatives or work coordinator, and everyday activities, such as cooking or laundering, may also reduce 'desocialization'. Mr Butler may need some support and training in some of these activities, such as laundry.

*Prognosis*

This cannot be accurately determined until a definite diagnosis is made and appropriate treatment begun. However, as Mr Butler recovered from two previous episodes, the prognosis for this episode is good, although the likelihood of recurrence is high. Mr Butler's deteriorating work history also suggests that despite symptomatic recovery, he may be becoming socially disabled.

## Further details

Mr Butler's parents saw the doctor on one occasion but they were reluctant to be involved in further interviews that seemed to them to be critically scrutinizing either their past or present family relationships.

More detailed historical information came to light in subsequent interviews with Mr Butler, however, and the effect of treatment and the passage of time also became apparent. He was next admitted a year later, initially as an inpatient for eight weeks, and then for 20 months as a day patient. His history, from the start of his illness up to his discharge at that time, is summarized below.

*History of presenting complaint*

Mr Butler first noticed that he was hard of hearing at the age of 20. This had not inconvenienced him until, as a result of promotion, he moved to a new open plan office in which there was a constant buzz of conversation. He had difficulty in hearing what was said to him, and social encounters became more and more of a strain. He took to drinking at lunchtimes before coming back to the office, and began to think the young girls in the office were discussing his sexual inadequacy and assumed that he was homosexual. He became preoccupied with his lack of previous sexual relationships and felt guilty about his previous sexual behaviour, for which he thought he could be prosecuted. He gradually became convinced that he was going to be prosecuted for sexual offences and that the police were collecting evidence. His arrest for drunkenness reinforced this belief.

Mr Butler gradually became depressed as his difficulties at work increased. He also began to feel increasingly 'cornered' by the police, which probably led to his suicide attempt. Both these feelings improved during his first two hospital admissions, but Mr Butler could not face going back to work and resigned. He obtained another, less responsible, job. However, after ten months he became convinced that situations at work were being set up by the police to test him, his drinking increased and he eventually left. He was unemployed for some time and gradually felt less 'cornered' by the police, although he spent an increasing amount of time in bed. Eventually he took another job but this lasted less time than the first and was closely followed by several other short-term jobs until he was again charged with being drunk and disorderly. After this Mr Butler stayed at home because 'the police are everywhere putting pressure on me'.

Mr Butler discharged himself during his third admission because he believed that the hospital staff were in league with the police.

The admission during which the original history was obtained occurred three months later. Mr Butler was treated with eight applications of electro-convulsive treatment (ECT), with risperidone and with fluoxetine. His mental state improved considerably but it was not clear which of these was the effective agent. He was not fully recovered on discharge: for example, although he no longer thought that the police were investigating him, he remained convinced they had done so in the past and might do so again.

Mr Butler was maintained in outpatients on risperidone and fluoxetine. After four months he found a job in an accounts department and said that he was enjoying it, despite having difficulty concentrating. Three months later, following an elective left stapedectomy, his left ear was temporarily plugged and his medication was withdrawn. He became convinced that the nurses were treating him particularly coldly, and that this was because he had insulted some nurses in a public house some years before.

His suspicion of the police also returned after his discharge and, a few days after returning to work, he walked out of his job. Risperidone was re-started and two months later Mr Butler was much less bothered about the police and work was again going well. The psychiatrist who was following him up gradually withdrew his medication, because he thought he had recovered. His suspicions flared up again, he began drinking regularly at lunchtime and in the evenings, and subsequently he left his work. After risperidone was re-started he felt well enough to get temporary employment. However, from the day this started he was sure that his colleagues knew of the police's interest in him and he only just managed to finish his two-week placement. A fortnight at another factory was even worse. Mr Butler's feelings of persecution fluctuated in intensity over the next two months. He was re-started on fluoxetine, and improved slightly after both the risperidone and fluoxetine were increased. One month later he felt himself to be as persecuted by the police and as guilty about his sexual misdemeanours as before, and 'on the brink of an overdose'. He was briefly admitted to hospital and was somewhat better on discharge, but still suspicious.

In the next few months Mr Butler spent more and more time in bed. He refused to allow his community nurse access to his residence and declined day-patient attendance but eventually wrote to the psychiatrist to describe 'the latest examples of police harassment', which included wiring his home to amplify the noise of traffic. He had taken, he wrote, to carrying a hammer 'to defend myself'. He was again admitted, and he confirmed he had not been taking his medication. The admitting psychiatrist noted that he was 'relaxed, not elated or depressed', even though he believed agents of the police were recording the interview. No other account of abnormal experiences was elicited.

Although Mr Butler's suspicions lessened on regular treatment with intramuscular depot fluphenazine he was noted to be withdrawn. He was referred to a day hospital where the admitting psychiatrist noted that, except for his ready smile, his face was unusually immobile and his tone of voice was monotonous. His answers to questions were unusually non-discursive. Mr Butler rarely volunteered new information, and was noted never to initiate conversations with other patients.

Mr Butler continued to receive intramuscular medication throughout his rehabilitation. He was very capable, particularly at clerical work, and so was given the patients' wages to prepare. However, in his first week of this he became convinced that a fellow patient was a plain-clothes policeman.

His suspicions subsided and four months later Mr Butler was transferred to a vocational resettlement where he was noted to be a conscientious worker but unusually slow and lacking in initiative. His suspiciousness was also remarked upon, and during this time he became increasingly convinced that there was a conspiracy against him to get information for the police or to test his masculinity; his account differed on various occasions. Eventually he refused to attend and he was referred to a day centre. At first he came in very late and often missed days unexpectedly, but his attendance gradually became more regular. He had several minor relapses, usually after being given more responsibility. One paranoid episode began in a pub after an unusually heavy bout of drinking when he believed that a woman who asked him for a light was testing his virility. These relapses were successfully managed with a temporary increase in medication and a reassessment of his work programme.

Mr Butler became engaged to a fellow patient about one year after starting at the day centre and, after an initial period of impotence, began a regular sexual relationship with his fiancée.

## Mental state examination

This was undertaken 18 months after his arrival at the day centre.

*Appearance and general behaviour*

Mr Butler was a markedly plump man who made no spontaneous movements. He had a mild Parkinsonian tremor when anxious. His voice was soft but normally modulated. His face was immobile except for occasional, self-deprecating smiles. His clothes were slightly unkempt and grubby.

*Speech*

He showed little spontaneity, and gave only brief, limited answers to direct questions. Often, at the end of an interview, he asked whether he was getting better.

*Mood*

Mr Butler was slightly tense but not depressed. He described himself as feeling 'fine'. He was attempting to diet to reduce weight.

*Thought content*

He was not thinking much about the police, although sometimes, when he remembered what had happened to him, he thought it 'funny' but did not like to think about it further. Mr Butler's mind generally appeared to be empty of any thoughts.

*Abnormal beliefs and interpretations of events*

Very occasionally he experienced an everyday scene as being of special significance to him but he paid little attention to it and quickly forgot it.

*Abnormal experiences*

None were elicited.

*Cognitive state*

Mr Butler's orientation, memory, concentration and attention were all normal.

*Self-appraisal*

He thought that he had had an illness but that his present inability to re-acclimatize to a work routine was due to 'laziness'.

## Reassessment

Mr Butler is a 39-year-old man with a 10-year history of a progressively incapacitating tendency to ideas of reference and persecutory beliefs that have recently rendered him incapable of open employment. The main challenge is to minimize the frequency of relapse of his illness. In order to achieve this the cause of relapse needs to be understood.

*Diagnosis*

Mr Butler's gradual social deterioration, punctuated by episodes typical of the 'positive' symptoms of schizophrenia, makes the diagnosis of schizophrenia certain. Since persecutory ideas continue to predominate, paranoid schizophrenia remains the correct sub-type.

*Aetiology*

These also have become rather clearer. Mr Butler's deafness, in combination with his lifelong shyness and social difficulties, probably contributed to the development of his schizophrenia as it did to his relapse when one ear was occluded following a stapedectomy. However, effective treatment of his deafness has not arrested the progress of his illness.

Mr Butler is a regular heavy drinker. He used alcohol to lower some of his social inhibitions and, as indicated by his heavy drinking at least at the start of his illness, to try and reduce his fear of imaginary persecution. Although there has been at least one occasion when heavy drinking precipitated the development of a persecutory delusion, which took some time to fade away, his normal steady intake appears not to exacerbate his illness.

The most important precipitants of relapse now seem to be, first, the expectation of an authority (such as the manager of the day centre) that he take on more responsible work and, second, withdrawal of his medication. However, expectations placed on him by his family and his fiancée may also be contributory factors.

### Further information

The major outstanding investigation is to see Mr Butler with his parents.

### Management

Mr Butler's long-term management has two goals: to minimize the dislocation and distress of relapse into positive symptoms and to help him attain as normal work and social relationships as possible.

Regular and consistent support is relevant to both these goals. The minimum dose of regular antipsychotic medication needs to be found which will keep his symptoms in abeyance. There also needs to be a pathway for him, his family and the manager at the day centre to the psychiatrist so that a rapid increase in medication can be given if this is needed; for example, during a recurrence of positive symptoms.

Outpatient sessions should also be used to encourage him in the appropriate amount of work and domestic activity to undertake and to monitor his progress in achieving his goals in these areas. Mr Butler is helped by encouragement and by being given a rationale for treatment. The manager at the day centre (and, possibly in the future, his family) can also be encouraged to maintain a realistic expectation of his achievements and helped in their disappointment if he fails to achieve his goals.

The nutritionist should prescribe an appropriate diet as his increasing weight may predispose him to medical problems and will only exacerbate his social anxiety. As medication is likely to have contributed to this, there is a further reason for keeping it to a minimum. Fluphenazine is no more likely than other neuroleptics to increase appetite, and a change of antipsychotic is therefore unlikely to be helpful.

Regular monitoring for the appearance of side effects, particularly tardive dyskinesia, should be instituted. Anticholinergic agents are often given, unnecessarily, to treat the side effects of long-term neuroleptics. They should therefore be avoided as they may increase the risk of dyskinesia.

*Prognosis*

Mr Butler is likely to remain socially disabled, although it can be expected that he will be free of his persecutory ideas most of the time. His mother has continued to supervise his appearance and self-care at home and to provide him with meals and clean clothes. He will probably continue to need some degree of daily supervision of this kind. He is unlikely to obtain open employment and would become socially isolated if he were not encouraged to attend a day centre.

The course of his illness cannot be predicted, but further deterioration can probably be prevented by the social interventions already mentioned. The risk of more severe deterioration is less than if Mr Butler had developed schizophrenia when he was younger, if he had not successfully established himself at work, and if he had a sub-type of schizophrenia other than 'paranoid'.

## Postscript

Mr and Mrs Butler senior eventually agreed to be seen with their son. Both expressed their grief at their son's deterioration. No one liked to talk about it at home. Mrs Butler's attitude to her son was critical but she was rarely firm with him; for example, about his helping out at home, or getting out of bed. Mr Butler kept out of his son's way. In an emotional moment he explained that if he behaved in a more concerned way he was afraid that his son would think that he was being treated as 'less than a man'. Both were very frightened when the doctor spoke of their son as 'disabled', but they also seemed relieved.

Possibly the most useful result of this meeting, which was not repeated, was that Mr Butler subsequently discussed his father's relentless appetite for work. When he retired on medical grounds his father had immediately taken another job that entailed him getting up at 4.30 in the morning. It was his son's inability to work that he and his son found so incomprehensible and disturbing about his illness. Mr Butler's wish to emulate his father seemed to explain Mr Butler's tendency to take on work that was beyond him and then to react to the consequent stress by becoming more and more convinced that he was being persecuted.

# Chapter 12

# A Panic Attack

## Mrs Woolfe

**Presenting complaint**

Mrs Woolfe attended with her cohabitee. Five weeks before her referral to the psychiatry outpatient department, Mrs Woolfe, while driving to work, experienced a sudden attack of severe anxiety. She described an initial feeling of foreboding followed by the rapid development of extreme fear, which was accompanied by sweating, palpitations, choking sensations and difficulty in breathing. The episode lasted about an hour. Since that time she had suffered many similar attacks, averaging two to three a day. Between episodes she was left feeling 'flat, tired and drained'. In the past three weeks she had also begun to feel low in her spirits and lacking in energy. She found herself brooding on thoughts of death and had horrifying images of harming herself or those close to her. She felt that her life was now hopeless and that there was nothing to live for. Her sleep was very disturbed and she had lost one stone (6 kg) in weight. Her concentration had become so impaired that she had stopped working two weeks earlier. Diazepam, 2mg three times daily, was prescribed by her general practitioner one week after the onset of her symptoms and this had provided some mild relief.

## Family history

Mrs Woolfe's father, aged 72, was a retired schoolmaster. She described him as 'one of the healthiest people I have known' until the last year, when he suffered a myocardial infarct. Although this was followed by a good physical recovery, he remained preoccupied with his health.

Her mother, aged 60, had 'suffered from nerves' all her life and she could not recall her ever being 'completely well'. She always seemed to be tense and preoccupied with trivial worries, and was frequently very low in her spirits. She often complained of physical symptoms, but her general practitioner was never able to make a clear-cut diagnosis and he usually prescribed 'bed rest'. She had always resisted referral to a psychiatrist, despite frequent suggestions by her general practitioner. Six months before, she had suffered a cerebrovascular accident with some speech and motor impairment, but had now fully recovered.

Mrs Woolfe was an only child. Her family was extremely religious and had attended church three times on Sundays; they considered it virtuous to forego all pleasures. Her parents' marriage was always very secure, conflict was rare and her mother was the dominant partner. Despite a very strict upbringing the patient had always felt close to both her parents and remembered feeling that she must not hurt them. People had, from an early age, commented on her over-developed sense of guilt when acting not in accordance with her parents' wishes. An uncle of her mother's had committed suicide, but she was unaware of the details because the matter was never discussed. There was no other family history of mental illness.

## Personal history

Mrs Woolfe's birth and early development were normal and her early childhood unremarkable. When she commenced school, aged five, she experienced some initial difficulty settling down. She was reluctant to attend at first and ran home on a few occasions. Her mother always took her back immediately and she soon became a happy primary school pupil. From 8 to 16 years she attended a private school and passed eight GCSEs. She made close friendships and was regarded by her teachers as a serious, hard-working girl. When she was 17 years old she was sent to a new school to study for her A levels. This school was very different from her previous one and she felt very unhappy there. She made no friends and was very upset by the fiercely competitive atmosphere. At this time she developed a number of symptoms (described under the past psychiatric history). Despite these difficulties she gained three A levels. Although she could have probably gone to university she chose to go to a secretarial college. After qualifying she worked as a secretary in a building society's legal department where she impressed the staff with her abilities and after a year there she began to work for a firm of solicitors where again she showed herself to be an extremely capable person. However, after two years she left to raise her family, and she did not work again for five years.

Seven years previously she began working at the head office of a publishing firm. Rapid promotion followed and at the time of her presentation she was in a senior managerial post bearing considerable responsibilities for organization and some of the legal aspects of the business. A month before the onset of her symptoms she had organized a large conference, which she found 'quite stressful'. She had also commenced an external university degree, of which she had completed two years.

She met her future husband, a stockbroker, when she was 16 years old and he was 26. They married three years later. They were married for 13 years until Mrs Woolfe left her husband one year ago. They had two children, an 11-year-old son and an 8-year-old daughter. Within a year or two of the marriage Mrs Woolfe began to feel that she had made a mistake. She described her husband as 'an overbearing man' who would never discuss things with her on an equal standing. Although he said he had wanted children he spent little time with them. She tried unsuccessfully to tell him of her dissatisfaction and suggested that they attend a marriage counsellor. This provoked arguments and he flatly refused, even after she told him of an affair. On occasions he had been violent, although never causing serious harm.

The couple finally separated, fairly amicably, one year previously. Mrs Woolfe went to live with her current cohabitee, Peter, who worked as an editor for the same firm. They had known each other for six years and had decided simultaneously to leave their spouses, he proving more reluctant, initially, than she. Her children lived with them but Peter's son was with the son's mother. About two months prior to Mrs Woolfe's attendance at the hospital, Peter began to feel miserable, particularly about his limited access to his son. He told her he had doubts about whether he could really love anyone again and decided that he would leave for two weeks 'to think it over'. It was after the first week that Mrs Woolfe developed her symptoms. Peter returned immediately and stated that his doubts were entirely resolved and that he wanted to carry on living with her.

## Previous personality

Mrs Woolfe was normally an energetic woman. She was efficient, orderly and reliable. She set high standards for herself, which she rarely felt she achieved. Although she was sociable and friendly, and coped well with strangers in the work situation, she did not have any close friends apart from Peter. Many people commented on her life-long tendency to devalue herself and to blame herself if others were unhappy. Although not religious she had a high moral code of behaviour. At times she felt miserable, but apart from one occasion (see below) this had not interfered with her ability to cope and she was not an excessive worrier. She had many interests including music, especially ballet, and collecting antique ceramics. She drank socially and was a non-smoker.

## Past medical history

There was no significant previous physical illness.

## Past psychiatric history

Although Mrs Woolfe had never seen a psychiatrist before, she described the development of clear-cut psychiatric symptoms when she was 17. This occurred when she changed school to do her A levels. During a play reading at school she developed her first attack of severe anxiety, the features of which were identical to those described earlier. She went on to develop a number of phobic symptoms as well, particularly of crowded places, buses and shops. These had become so intense that she was unable to attend school for about six weeks. Gradually, with the help of her general practitioner and her parents, who encouraged her to go out, she improved over one year. During that time she recalled feeling quite depressed.

Since that time she had remained almost completely symptom-free, apart from occasional apprehension of travelling on the Underground.

## Mental state examination

### Appearance and general behaviour

Mrs Woolfe was a petite, slim lady who, when the interview commenced, said that she was too anxious to speak and suggested that Peter be called in to give an account of her problems. She appeared very anxious and complained of sweating palms and of feeling breathless. At times she was tearful, particularly when describing her more distressing symptoms.

### Speech

After some initial reassurance she was able to give a well organized and fluent account of herself and required little prompting.

### Mood

She described a depressed mood. She felt 'worn out, incompetent and hopeless; however hard I try I'm just not going to get better…there's just a terrible, terrible sadness – a sort of continual hurt inside'. On direct questioning she admitted to some fleeting suicidal thoughts but she did not feel that things had reached 'that point yet'. She had no appetite and had lost over a stone in weight in five weeks. Her sleep was poor, with initial insomnia and early morning waking (3 or 4 a.m.). She described a marked diurnal variation in her mood, feeling at her worst first thing in the morning and better by the early afternoon. Her depressed mood was sustained without even a moment's relief and she found no pleasure in anything.

*Thought content*

A number of preoccupations emerged. She was terrified of her panic attacks. These consisted of an intense experience of fear and were accompanied by the somatic symptoms previously described. She feared that she might die during one of these attacks. She also described extremely distressing, vivid, stereotyped, recurrent images, usually of harming herself or those close to her, such as stabbing herself with a kitchen knife. She attempted to push these intrusive images out of her mind and she feared that she might act them out although she did not wish to. Mrs Woolfe also described a number of guilt-laden ruminations, particularly about having abandoned her husband and about being a burden on her parents and Peter. She said that she had let her parents down badly, although conceding that they had supported her separation from her husband and that they liked Peter. She denied any fears that Peter would now leave her and she described him in the kindest terms.

She had no current phobic symptoms.

*Abnormal beliefs and interpretations of events*

No delusions or hallucinations were elicited. Her ideas of guilt and hopelessness were not of delusional intensity and she had no hypochondriacal preoccupations.

*Abnormal experiences*

Mrs Woolfe described no abnormal experiences, in particular no symptoms of depersonalization or derealization.

*Cognitive state*

Cognitive testing revealed her to be well orientated and without any signs of memory impairment. She was able to concentrate well enough to perform 'serial sevens' without difficulty, although she had complained that her concentration was impaired to the extent that she could not look at a newspaper or watch even a short television programme.

*Self-appraisal*

Mrs Woolfe did not readily accept that she was ill and at one point said there was nothing that could change her and she was therefore wasting the doctor's valuable time. 'There are surely many more needy people than me; the responsibility for my state lies with me.'

## Physical examination

The general practitioner had performed a physical examination before referring Mrs Woolfe to the psychiatrist and this had revealed no abnormality.

Peter was seen after Mrs Woolfe had been interviewed. He confirmed the history in every detail and described her personality before her illness in similar terms to her own.

## Preliminary assessment

Mrs Woolfe is a 32-year-old woman who has separated from her husband and recently had a brief separation from her cohabitee. Following this she has felt panicky, anxious, and more recently, depressed. This type of problem is frequently met in outpatients, where the psychiatrist needs to reach a clear diagnosis in order to start treatment. In this case the important diagnostic issues are whether her symptoms reflect primarily a depressive or an anxiety-based disturbance, or whether it should be accepted as a 'normal' response to her situation.

*Diagnosis*

Mrs Woolfe's presentation is dominated by symptoms of anxiety and depression. The major possibilities to be considered are a depressive illness, an anxiety state or an adjustment reaction.

Most of the symptoms typical of an anxiety state are present. These include subjective anxiety with somatic accompaniments (sweating, palpitations, choking sensations, difficulty in breathing) that typically occur in panic attacks. Her anxiety is diffuse and not focused on any particular situation or object. The short duration of the symptoms is also consistent with this diagnosis. However, there are also a number of severe depressive symptoms, which tend to dominate the mental state examination. An admixture of depressive symptoms in patients with an anxiety state is common but generally less marked than here. The onset of an anxiety state is usually, but not always, in association with a precipitating factor. In this case, the onset of her symptoms coincided with the departure of Mrs Woolfe's cohabitee to think about their relationship.

The presence of clear-cut depressive symptoms leads to a depressive illness as the primary diagnosis. She describes a sustained depressed mood, lack of energy, poor concentration, a feeling of hopelessness that she will never change, ideas of guilt about abandoning her husband, letting down her parents, being a burden on those she loves, and being responsible for her current state and therefore of wasting the psychiatrist's time. She also has the so-called 'biological' features of depression, appetite disturbance and weight loss, early morning waking and diurnal mood variation. In addition she admits to fleeting suicidal ideas. The terrifying visual images of harming herself or others are obsessional in nature, in that they were unwanted, intrusive, stereotyped mental contents that she attempted to resist and which she perceived as alien to her personality and inappropriate. Their content was morbid and depressive. Obsessional symptoms of this type are common in depressive illnesses. Anxiety symptoms are also common in depressive illness although they do not usually stand out as starkly as in this case. The combination of depression and tension in Mrs Woolfe might warrant a description of agitated depression.

The third possibility to be considered is an 'adjustment reaction'. This is a mild or transient disturbance that is usually closely related in time and content to an obvious stressful event. Mrs Woolfe's symptoms developed in close relationship to Peter leaving. However, the extent of her disturbance, and its failure to improve when he returned, suggests that this was more than an adjustment reaction. With time her symptoms of depression have intensified. Furthermore, the content of her depressive and anxious preoccupations are not directly related to the separation. An element that should also be considered is an individual's vulnerability to this type of stress. She has suffered psychological distress twice previously, both at times of major changes in her life. The first, when she started school, was apparently mild and transient, whereas the second, when she changed school to study for her A level examinations, was prolonged and severe, and comprised a mixture of depression and anxiety symptoms, the latter taking the form of panic attacks and agoraphobia. The second episode, as in the present illness, appears to have been too long-lived and severe to be termed an adjustment reaction. Between the ages of 18 and 33 Mrs Woolfe coped well with many stresses and there is no evidence of major disruptions of her life.

Overall, the most likely diagnosis is of a depressive illness. There is the possibility that this is Mrs Woolfe's second depressive illness, the first having occurred when she was 17 years old.

*Aetiology*

There is a family history of mental disorder. Mrs Woolfe's mother has had life-long problems of a psychological kind, possibly with depressive and anxiety symptoms. Also, her mother's uncle committed suicide, raising the possibility that he might have suffered from a severe depressive illness. The transmission of a psychiatric disorder from mother to daughter could be by genetic or learning influences or a combination of both.

In the year prior to the development of her illness, Mrs Woolfe experienced an astonishing number of stressful life events. She left her husband to live with another man, her father had a heart attack, her mother had a stroke, she was promoted at work, and finally Peter left home. There is a relationship between life events and the onset of illnesses of many kinds. In general the type of life event does not have a specific relationship with the type of illness that ensues, although 'losses', defined broadly, are often associated with depressive symptoms. Usually the type of illness bears a closer relationship to the patient's particular vulnerabilities, which in turn are linked to 'constitutional' factors (in which genetics, for example, may play a role), and past experiences.

Mrs Woolfe is an intelligent and capable woman who, from the information available, appears to be of a reasonably stable disposition, at least since her late teens. There are, however, some aspects of her personality that might have made it especially difficult for her to manage some of the life changes she experienced. A theme running through her life has been a special sensitivity to her very religious parents and a propensity for feeling guilty if others should feel disappointed or unhappy. Her parents had a strict code of conduct and Mrs Woolfe expressed a loyalty to it. Leaving her husband to live with another man followed by the development of serious illnesses in both parents might be expected to affect Mrs Woolfe with special force. Peter's leaving may then have spelled the final disappointment and sign of failure in re-establishing her life that might have compensated for leaving her husband. Less important, although possibly of significance, might have been her rapid promotion at work, which entailed new responsibilities. This is likely to have proved particularly stressful for a person like Mrs Woolfe, who sets high standards, is conscientiousness and needs to be in control. These life-long perfectionist traits are not sufficiently prominent to warrant the description of 'obsessional'.

The content of many of Mrs Woolfe's preoccupations in her illness can be seen to derive from some of the central themes in her life: guilt at letting others down, being a burden on her close ones, harming her close ones and incompetence.

### Further information

At this stage there is sufficient information to make a diagnosis and to plan the initial treatment, especially since Peter has been interviewed and has substantiated the history provided by Mrs Woolfe.

It would be useful to know more about the family history of mental disorder and whether her mother and her mother's uncle had suffered from depressive illness. The family doctor might be able to provide useful information here.

The stability of Mrs Woolfe's relationship with Peter and their hopes for the future need some exploration and this could be done in a joint session with the couple. It is not clear that seeing Mrs Woolfe's parents at this stage would add any important information.

## Management

Mrs Woolfe presents with a moderately severe depressive illness that may still be getting worse. The question of admission to hospital needs to be considered, particularly as she has entertained some suicidal thoughts and will need considerable supervision and support.

During the interview Mrs Woolfe eventually made a good rapport and she appeared to speak openly about her feelings with no attempt at concealment. Peter expressed a wish to look after her and they both agreed that her parents could also be enlisted to help. Admission is likely to be unnecessary. It is important at this stage to explain to Mrs Woolfe and Peter that she is suffering from a depressive illness from which she will almost certainly recover. It might also prove helpful to reassure her about the nature of some of her symptoms; in particular that she will not die from her panic attacks and that she will not act on her obsessional impulses. To be effective, explanation and reassurance require the establishment of a good doctor–patient relationship and this must be an immediate and major goal.

Antidepressant medication is indicated and paroxetine would be suitable because it is also useful in panic disorder. The anticipated delay in the response to medication should be mentioned, as should possible side effects. In view of the seriousness of the illness she should be seen weekly initially, in order to monitor the effectiveness of the medication, to intervene if her condition should deteriorate and to provide continuing support for her and Peter until she improves.

The longer-term management will depend on Mrs Woolfe's response to medication. It is to be expected that she will improve over the next month or so. As long as her improvement is maintained simple psychological support should suffice. If significant problems in her relationship with Peter emerge these might be tackled in joint interviews when the depression has improved.

## Prognosis

The prognosis for recovery from this episode is excellent. The acute onset with clear-cut depressive symptoms marking a radical change from the patient's normal self augur a good response to medication. Mrs Woolfe is a woman with many personality assets and she should be able to resume her normal life. There remains the possibility that she may have further episodes of depression, particularly as this may now be her second illness. Such an episode is most likely to occur if she is exposed to mounting pressures.

## Further details

Following discussion, Mrs Woolfe indicated that she would be prepared to take medication although she did not see that it could possibly help.

Over the next three months she did well. She was seen weekly for a while and then fortnightly. The dose of paroxetine was increased to 30mg and her depressive and anxiety symptoms diminished markedly. Peter appeared concerned and supportive. Problems between the couple were consistently denied, and evidence of their existence did not emerge in two joint sessions. After six weeks' leave, Mrs Woolfe returned to work. She was somewhat lacking in confidence but managed to cope well. After three months she was discharged from the clinic. She remained somewhat troubled by very occasional panic attacks and the fear that her depression might recur. Her general practitioner was advised to continue her medication for another three months and then to tail it off.

Nine months after her original presentation Mrs Woolfe was referred back to the clinic. Many of her symptoms had recurred but had not reached their previous intensity. Paroxetine had been stopped two months previously. Two new events had also occurred: the offer of a divorce from her husband and the need to organize a large conference for her firm.

The psychiatrist decided that Mrs Woolfe was having a relapse of her depressive illness, probably because her medication had been stopped prematurely. However, on this occasion another observation was made. Although Mrs Woolfe responded strikingly to reassurance from the doctor, Peter seemed unable to comfort her at all. Whenever the psychiatrist mentioned the couple's relationship, or made any reference to Peter's leaving, it was always avoided by a shift to another topic. At these times Mrs Woolfe and Peter looked away from each other. There was a sense that all was not well with the couple and he suggested they be seen together for a few sessions in order to understand this more.

Paroxetine was recommenced and again Mrs Woolfe improved gradually. During the joint sessions it was striking how protective of each other the couple were. They seemed at pains not to distress each other and any hint of disagreement, when taken up by the doctor, was quickly detoured to a discussion of Mrs Woolfe's symptoms. At times Peter uttered some quite depressive thoughts, mainly concerning his son whom he felt he had let down by leaving his wife. These were quickly covered up, usually by Mrs Woolfe saying this was understandable and only temporary.

Three months after her return to the clinic she attended alone. She had been unable to persuade Peter to come and said he had become listless and uncommunicative, and was ruminating excessively about his son. He was unwilling to discuss his feelings with her. She admitted for the first time that these spells had occurred frequently, particularly in the first six months of their cohabitation. At these times she felt helpless in her attempts to influence his mood. The doctor suggested Mrs Woolfe try and encourage Peter to return.

The next time she attended with a female friend. Peter had left her and had gone to live with his parents. His wife had remarried and he had become extremely depressed. He had also expressed some vague persecutory ideas concerning people at work. Her friend said that Peter had been inclined to depressive moods all along and that Mrs Woolfe had struggled to prop him up. Mrs Woolfe admitted for the first time that she had been very concerned about Peter, even from the commencement of their cohabitation. There had been weekends when he stayed in bed for practically the entire time, not bothering to wash or eat and 'engrossed in his own thoughts to which he denied me access'. On one occasion he expressed some bizarre ideas about the bedroom light, which he felt 'was spying' on his thoughts and behaviour. She had 'hugged him like a child to comfort him'. In the view of her friend, the couple had never succeeded in establishing any 'sense of family' in their home.

Although Mrs Woolfe was distressed by Peter leaving, this had a quality, different in kind, from her previous state of depression. Her reaction felt normal and it seemed as if a burden had been eased. It became clear how troubling the relationship had been for her, particularly Peter's imperviousness to her attempts to make him feel better. She was someone who needed to see her efforts rewarded in order to feel worthwhile. Her sense of loyalty to him had prevented her from disclosing this earlier.

## Reassessment

Although Peter has left Mrs Woolfe following her relapse, she seems to have improved. The context of her depression has now changed and the original assessment needs to be reconsidered in order to take account of this. In particular, understanding why she first became depressed will shape any further treatment.

### Diagnosis

The original diagnosis remains depression. Mrs Woolfe has suffered a subsequent relapse, but has now improved.

### Aetiology

It seems possible that the withdrawal of medication contributed to Mrs Woolfe's relapse. Her first episode of depression, when she was 17, had lasted for one year. The advice about when to discontinue medication had not taken into account the possibility that this might have been the natural time course of her illness.

Mrs Woolfe had also been given responsibility for organizing another conference. A similar event occurred a month before her original presentation and it seems likely that this has again contributed to her relapse.

Although the offer of a divorce from her husband might have been expected and wanted, it would also have been stressful; not only because it finalized their separation, but also because of its impact upon her relationship with Peter. She would have been in a position to remarry and might have felt emotional pressure to do so. In the light of what has been discovered about Peter this would have been a considerable source of worry.

Peter's seriously disturbed behaviour was clearly an important factor contributing to Mrs Woolfe's depression. Living with him was a continuous source of stress and since this was never revealed to the psychiatrist he was unable to provide any counselling about this situation. Both Peter and Mrs Woolfe had actively avoided bringing his problem to the psychiatrist, in spite of ample encouragement. This seems surprising considering the strain it must have imposed upon their relationship. Although Peter might have been reluctant to discuss this because he was feeling persecuted, there may have been reasons for Mrs Woolfe to avoid this issue, too.

Her sense of guilt when others are unhappy might have made her feel that she must try and sort out Peter's problems on her own. Furthermore, there are similarities between Peter and the way she described her first husband. In particular they were both unable to share and work out problems with her, as she would have liked. It is not uncommon for people to develop relationships with a recurring pattern of this nature that often seem to reflect some difficulty of their own. The fact that Mrs Woolfe might have felt that she had made the same mistake twice is probably sufficient reason for not drawing anyone's attention to it. There were also similarities between Mrs Woolfe's problem and Peter's, in particular their feeling of guilt about a broken marriage. It is again not uncommon for someone to find a partner who has similar problems.

These factors suggest how Mrs Woolfe might have been drawn into a distressing relationship with Peter and the reasons why she might have found it difficult to discuss this with the psychiatrist. It now seems clearer how her depression developed and was maintained. It also seems likely that aspects of her personality made her particularly susceptible to develop such a relationship in the first place.

## Further information

The likelihood that aspects of her personality have made her vulnerable to depression means that these need to be clarified. For example, she appears to develop relationships with men who are unable to discuss their problems with her. She then tries hard to support them, whilst resenting their inability to share experiences with her. Mrs Woolfe could be invited to reflect upon whether this is a recurring pattern in her relationships by asking her to consider ways in which she felt she might have contributed to any of the difficulties that existed. A clearer picture of her vulnerability to depression should then emerge. Her capacity to respond to this style of discussion will also convey whether she would be able to make use of this information within the framework of a psychotherapeutic relationship.

## Management

Mrs Woolfe will continue to require antidepressant medication because of the severity of her symptoms and their tendency to recur. These should be withdrawn under supervision only after she has made a sustained recovery of at least six months. Increasing attention should be directed towards psychotherapeutic interventions, which will involve clarification of those issues which have been mentioned.

## Prognosis

She again appears to have made a good recovery from the immediate episode. Her vulnerability to relapse is likely to depend on the quality of future relationships, which will depend in part on her response to psychotherapy.

## Postscript

The psychiatrist continued Mrs Woolfe's antidepressant medication and saw her every month in the outpatient department. Although Peter did not return she often talked about him and expressed considerable doubt about her ability to live without a man. The psychiatrist focused on her lack of self-confidence and responded by being supportive and reassuring. He reminded her of her strengths, whilst also providing her with the opportunity to discuss her self-doubt. Her own resources, as well as the support that was forthcoming from her parents and old friends, surprised her. During the following year she carried on with her work and suffered no recurrence of her depressive symptoms. She had not embarked on a new relationship.

# Chapter 13

# I've Felt Different All My Life

## Miss Jordash

### Presenting complaint

Miss Jordash, a 32-year-old woman, attended the outpatient department accompanied by her partner. She said she had asked her general practitioner to make the referral because 'I feel I have got as far as I can go with him'. She had recently asked him to arrange for her to be admitted to hospital in order to escape from her 'day to day suffering'. Although she had felt unwell for most of her life, this seemed to have worsened over the last year and she was now experiencing 'morbid thoughts' and feeling extremely unhappy.

Miss Jordash said, 'I've felt different all of my life, because I've never fitted in with what other people expect of me.' Whereas she used to be able to cope with this, she now found it increasingly difficult. On many occasions over the years she had thought about harming herself by taking an overdose or by cutting herself. These thoughts were always impulsive, occurred when she was feeling 'low and fed up' and were generally precipitated by difficulties between her and her partner.

Her problems began around the time of menarche, when she was at secondary school. She had always felt more comfortable spending her time alone. She had joined a local swimming club, taken up long distance swimming, and swam up to three miles a day. This made her feel better, and even 'high'. However, she was only ever mediocre at the sport and did not enjoy competitions. Her parents disapproved of her level of involvement and this led to arguments at home. With regular exercise her weight began to drop and at its lowest point was about five and a half stone (she was about five feet tall). At this point in her life she began to avoid food, to eat less than one regular meal a day, and to make herself vomit. She became amenorrhoeic at the age of 15, which lasted until she was about 20. At this time she also suffered from constipation and began abusing laxatives that she obtained from her general practitioner and 'over the counter'. Her weight remained constantly low until she was 23 years old when she commenced lithium therapy and it rose to its present level of about eight and a half stone.

Miss Jordash had suffered from 'morbid thoughts' from her early teens. These were intrusive, unwanted images, which she recognized as the product of her own mind. They usually involved some traumatic accident occurring to someone close to her. For example, she would see her partner fall in front of a car, or her son, Connor, fall from a slide. The thoughts were short-lived and led to feelings of anxiety, which she tried to resist. Their occurrence seemed to be related to her mood and stressors in her life at the time.

She first tried to harm herself after an argument at home with her brother, when she was nine years old. Both her parents worked, so her older brother looked after her for significant periods of time. At that time she remembered feeling abandoned and unloved, and that her brother was 'bossy and controlling'.

Her first overdose 'probably' occurred when she was 20. She was still living with her parents at the time and felt unhappy with both her home and her work. She had taken a 'handful of aspirins' in front of some friends, because she felt they were ignoring her. They subsequently made her vomit. Since then this had happened on numerous occasions, 'too many to remember'. At least three or four of the episodes had been 'serious' and resulted in her attending a local Accident and Emergency centre, where she had a stomach washout and had to take activated charcoal. On two occasions she was admitted for further medical supervision and transferred to a psychiatric unit. A typical overdose consisted of her impulsively taking 'handfuls of any medication that I could get hold of'. They were never planned or accompanied by a written note, and she did not think she had ever made a determined effort to kill herself. More recently, when this happened, she would sometimes inform a friend or a therapist about it later.

From the age of '25 or even earlier' Miss Jordash engaged in superficial self-laceration. She generally used a broken glass or a razor blade on her stomach and forearms, sometimes writing words such as 'ugly'. She felt this made her feel 'less tense'. This was now happening less than once a month, and she had reduced it principally for the sake of her son. On two occasions, when hospitalized, she had tried to strangle herself, but she was unable to remember further details.

At the present time Miss Jordash was managing to maintain a reasonably healthy diet. She was not bingeing or restricting her intake of food, and only occasionally used senna tablets, which were prescribed by her general practitioner. Her menstruation had returned, but was irregular, and she was swimming on a daily basis, but not for excessive distances.

Miss Jordash said her mood had fluctuated dramatically over the years, although most of the time she felt low. She had a chronic and pervasive feeling of being trapped in every aspect of her life and was dissatisfied with her position, her relationships and her job situation. She said, 'I have never really felt satisfied with life.' Her sleep pattern was variable, with initial insomnia and occasional waking in the night. She eventually wakes up at about 7.30 a.m. and gets on with her domestic chores. She described her current energy levels as 'good', her concentration as 'fair' and her libido as 'variable'.

## Family history

Miss Jordash was the younger of two siblings. Both her parents were aged 64 and well. Her father was a retired administrator and her mother worked in an accounts department of a local firm. Her elder brother was aged 35 and worked in finance. No one else in her family had similar problems or had seen a psychiatrist. However, she said she knew her mother had experienced mood swings and been treated with antidepressants by her general practitioner. Nevertheless, she felt all her family was very dismissive of psychiatric illness and hated the stigmatization associated with it.

## Personal history

She was born in Stoke-on-Trent, where she had lived all her life. While pregnant with Miss Jordash her mother suffered from elevated blood pressure and had to be hospitalized for long periods.

She described her parents as 'loving and caring'. However, they both worked very hard and she remembered feeling 'abandoned' by them, because they left home early to go to work and returned late.

Miss Jordash said an episode occurred in her childhood when 'I was made to feel very dirty'. She was only able to say, 'Something happened in a greenhouse with my brother and some of his friends.' She said she could not remember anything else and obviously found it very distressing to talk about.

She attended a secondary school until she was 16 and always felt a 'nervous wreck'. She had trouble reading and required extra lessons. She was also frequently bullied, had few close friends and became involved in a number of fights. She hated puberty. However, there were no significant discipline problems and she obtained four O levels and ten CSEs. After leaving school she began working for a local building firm as a secretary. She said 'the job was all right', but her female colleagues were 'bitchy'. As a result of this she resigned and took a job in another building firm, where she met her current partner. Her work was 'boring, tedious and stressful' and she found the management 'unforgiving'. She thought her female colleagues would not accept her and felt under pressure most of the time. She often argued with her colleagues and was asked to go home on one occasion, when she shouted at them. She had not really worked for the last nine years or so.

Miss Jordash's partner was a site manager for a firm of builders and they did not seem to have any financial problems. They met at work, started to live together after two years and had one son, Connor, now aged six. She described their relationship as 'constantly up and down' due to his drinking problems. This was now, apparently, currently under control. Connor attended a local primary school and she had been told he had 'learning difficulties'. He had few friends and she said he often hit himself with his school bag. He had been referred to a local child psychologist for assessment.

## Past medical history

Miss Jordash said she suffered from 'breathing problems and asthma'. The referral letter noted that she attended her general practice frequently, complaining of 'multiple, relatively trivial physical symptoms'.

At the time of referral Miss Jordash was taking paroxetine, 20mg once a day, becotide and ventolin for reversible airways disease, and diazepam, up to 5mg, when required. She said she took this less than once a week. She was unaware of any allergies. She did not smoke or use illicit drugs, and although she described past episodes of binge drinking, which were frequently followed by an overdose, she was now drinking less than once a week, and only minimal amounts.

## Past psychiatric history

Her first psychiatric admission occurred when she was 24 years old, shortly after she met her partner and had just bought a home. At that time both of them were out of work and she thought his drinking had caused the problems that led to her admission. According to her general practitioner the admission was for 'depression and suicidal ideation' and lasted about six weeks. Although she was initially a voluntary patient she was later detained under a section of the Mental Health Act, because she tried to leave. Following Connor's birth, a year later, she was admitted to a Mother and Baby Unit, again with depression and suicidal ideation. On this occasion she was treated with a course of ECT and, following discharge, she remained well for a short period of time.

There had been several other admissions for similar symptoms, but Miss Jordash was unable to remember the details. Two years previously she had completed a six-month course of cognitive behavioural psychotherapy that focused on a problem-solving approach. When asked whether it had been helpful she replied, 'All right.' Since then she had seen her general practitioner about every two weeks.

## Previous personality

As described, Miss Jordash had felt throughout her life that there was something wrong with her, certainly since puberty. She had always been an unhappy person who found it difficult to establish and maintain enjoyable and rewarding relationships.

## Mental state examination

### Appearance and general behaviour

Miss Jordash was a well-presented young woman of average build with medium-length brown hair, which covered her face at times. She appeared settled during the interview, but hardly smiled and was tearful when discussing emotional issues.

### Speech

She spoke fluently and coherently, at a normal rate and volume.

### Mood

Miss Jordash seemed slightly tense but was not overtly agitated. She felt 'low and mixed up', she described constantly wanting to change things in order to feel happier and she made it clear that she felt chronically dissatisfied with her life. She wanted to feel satisfied with her partner and Connor, as well as with herself, but had never really done so. Although she was self-evidently very unhappy, this was long-standing and she had not experienced any of the changes in her sleep or appetite that would suggest a major depression. She also said she had no thoughts about harming herself at the present time. Although she could not think of how her situation might improve she was not prepared to give up hope.

### Thought content

She described intrusive and unwanted morbid thoughts, as described above. Most of the time she also felt that she deserved to be punished, but could not understand why.

*Abnormal beliefs and interpretations of events*

She had always felt that people, particularly women, did not like her. However, she recognized this might have something to do with the way she felt about herself.

*Abnormal experiences*

She described hearing 'voices' inside her head. These spoke directly to her and were always critical. She thought they represented what she felt about herself and she tried to put them out of her mind.

*Cognitive state*

Her orientation, attention, and recall were normal. Her retention of a short address was good, although she performed less well on serial subtraction. She seemed of above average intelligence.

*Self-appraisal*

She expressed some curiosity about the cause of her discomfort, but was apathetic about the opportunity for change and had agreed to come and see a psychiatrist mainly because her partner had insisted.

## Physical examination

A physical examination was not carried out on this occasion.

## Preliminary assessment

Miss Jordash is a 32-year-old, unemployed, white woman with a young son. She has a ten-year history of contact with psychiatric services typified by episodes of low mood, suicidal ideation and impulsive self-harm. She has previously been detained under the Mental Health Act and treated with ECT. She gives a life-long description of conflictual relationships and describes chronic feelings of dissatisfaction with herself and others, including her carers.

## Diagnosis

Some of Miss Jordash's symptoms are compatible with depression: her low self-esteem, ideas of unworthiness, a bleak view of the future, ideas of self-harm and disturbed sleep. However, at the present time the picture is one of chronicity, with a consistent sense of dissatisfaction. The episodes of self-harm appear to have been largely in reaction to environmental stressors and in order to relieve anxiety, rather than to end her life. However, these may be confounded by fewer, but more serious, attempts to commit suicide, when she has been significantly depressed. Although she does not appear to be suffering from a major depressive episode at present, she may have in the past. This should become clearer when the details of previous admissions are available.

An alternative diagnosis is dysthymia. This is used to describe a long-standing low mood that is rarely severe enough to fulfil the criteria for depression.

Miss Jordash's life-long unhappiness first emerged during her adolescence and has been associated with considerable personal and social disruption. Her behaviour is maladaptive to a broad range of personal and social situations. These are the defining criteria for a diagnosis of personality disorder. This is a contentious diagnostic issue, partly because it lacks specificity since many of the characteristics are found in successful healthy individuals. The diagnosis of personality disorder has been criticized for being used to categorize individuals who are perceived as difficult and do not conform to societal norms. Miss Jordash's difficulties are characterized by her disturbed self-image, her chronic feelings of emptiness, her liability to become involved in intense, unstable relationships and a series of suicidal threats or acts of self-harm. These fulfil the criteria required for the diagnosis of emotionally unstable personality disorder of a borderline type (ICD10), or borderline personality disorder (DSMIV).

The second-person auditory phenomena she described may suggest the possibility of a psychotic element. However, further questioning clarified that these were only ever experienced inside her head and that she recognized them as a product of her own mind. It is therefore likely that they represent an increased awareness of her thinking, rather than hallucinatory activity.

*Aetiology*

Although a definite diagnosis has not yet been made, a number of factors could be significant. Her mother has been treated with antidepressants and may have experienced mood swings, which suggests a possible family history of affective disorder. There is some genetic contribution to depressive disorder, albeit rather less than to schizophrenia or bipolar disorder.

There is a contradiction in the manner in which she describes a loving and caring environment whilst she was growing up, but felt abandoned when her parents went to work early or returned late. This is consistent with a poor early attachment to her family, which is said to be indicative of later emotional difficulties, especially depression.

She described, with obvious distress, an episode involving her brother and possibly his friends, where she felt 'dirty'. This must raise the possibility of child sexual abuse. However, even if it represents a memory of normal childhood curiosity, retrospectively biased by her depressive attitude, the event clearly holds considerable meaning for her. It is difficult, and inappropriate, to open up these matters at the beginning of an interview. Further discussion should therefore be deferred until later and preferably reserved until later meetings, by when sufficient trust has developed.

Miss Jordash had difficult relationships with both her peers at school and her female colleagues at work. It may be useful to acquire more information about the precise nature of these interpersonal difficulties; whether she felt they were too distant or she had intense emotional attachments that did not survive her expectations. As a result of these difficulties she has discontinued working and felt unable to return. The absence of a role outside her home, or a structure to her day, is very likely to be reinforcing her current dissatisfaction, because she valued her work and it offered her the opportunity to improve her self-esteem.

There are further difficulties within her family that will have also reduced her self-esteem and have contributed to her feelings of depression. She has said her relationship with her partner is a source of conflict; in particular that he drinks excessively and that this precipitates arguments. The fact that her son is said to have learning difficulties would also serve to undermine Miss Jordash's self-esteem. When someone is depressed they feel responsible for the 'bad' things that happen around them. If Miss Jordash feels some responsibility for her son's difficulties and the friction within her relationship, this would be an example of what cognitive therapists refer to as 'negative thinking'.

Finally, cycles of social dysfunction commonly run in families, so that the parents' difficulties are perpetuated in their children by so-called inter-generational cycles.

### Further information

It would be helpful to see her partner alone, in order to provide a corroborative account of Miss Jordash's history and to clarify any current difficulties. In particular, he could confirm her son's health and comment on how they get along with each other. An assessment at home would provide an excellent opportunity to evaluate the quality of how she and Connor interact.

It is vital to obtain the medical records of Miss Jordash's previous inpatient episodes, to confirm the details of her previous presentations and assessments.

### Management

Pharmacotherapeutic interventions in the past seem to have achieved little except a short-term reduction in Miss Jordash's level of agitation. Her current antidepressant is an appropriate choice and is relatively safe should she take it in overdose.

Miss Jordash has a good relationship with her general practitioner, who is probably the first professional she has learned to trust and who offers an important role in maintaining stability for her. As far as possible any changes in her therapeutic relationships should be undertaken slowly in order to avoid destabilizing her condition.

There are specialized national services for patients with personality disorder and it may well be worthwhile considering a referral to this service for an assessment for residential management and support.

Further management will depend on a more precise determination of diagnosis and aetiology. She should be offered regular outpatient sessions to continue her assessment and to provide ongoing support. This will clarify her suitability for psychotherapy or referral to a more specialized residential unit.

*Prognosis*

This cannot be accurately determined until a definite diagnosis is made and appropriate treatment begun. However, Miss Jordash's difficulties have been lifelong and the outcome for individuals with borderline personality disorder is fair, at best. On the positive side, she has managed to maintain her relationship, despite the difficulties, and she has already changed some of her behaviour in order to protect her son. Her relationships could therefore be important in maintaining her motivation for change. Similarly, the life trajectory of this type of personality disorder is to ameliorate with age. Any depressive episodes should be treated aggressively in order to reduce their severity and length. However, even if she responds positively to these interventions, she will remain vulnerable to further episodes because of her sensitivity to external stressors and her difficulty in coping with change.

## Past psychiatric history

When she was 25 years old Miss Jordash began individual psychotherapy, which lasted 18 months. During the psychotherapy she had one further inpatient episode, when she alternated between being aggressive to staff and cutting herself. The staff found it extremely difficult to contain her behaviour safely so she was eventually sectioned and transferred to a locked ward.

A year later she was readmitted with severe depression and suicidal ideation. During this admission she apparently requested, and received, a course of ECT.

Miss Jordash's inpatient stays were typified by variability in her mental state, with intermittent episodes of agitation and aggression. On one occasion she required a high level of nursing observation, because she was threatening to harm herself. During periods of leave she returned to the ward either with her medication and threatening to take an overdose, or with a razor blade and threatening to lacerate herself. During one admission she climbed onto a second-storey fire escape and threatened to throw herself off, but was persuaded to come down by nursing staff.

Through the course of her admissions and outpatient treatment she had been prescribed a wide variety of minor and major tranquillizers, anti-depressants and mood-stabilizing drugs. None of these, either alone or in combination, had produced any sustained improvement in her condition.

When she was 28 years old she was referred for a specialist opinion. The detailed review concluded, 'Miss Jordash suffers from a borderline personality disorder with recurrent depressive episodes. She has significant and recurrent interpersonal difficulties, which are the main source of her problems. Medication is unlikely to be helpful in the longer term, and should only be used for short periods in order to alleviate specific symptoms.' Referral to a specialized day hospital service 'for psychological work' was recommended.

One year later, after a further assessment, she was admitted to the day hospital for treatment. During the course of this admission she was diagnosed as suffering from recurrent depression and an emotionally unstable personality disorder, borderline type. It was suggested she commence meclobemide, an antidepressant, in addition to their psychotherapeutic interventions. However, she found it difficult to settle in the unit and took increasing periods of leave. Eventually, after about two months, she discharged herself.

Since then she had only two further, brief, admissions. The first occurred probably when she was moving house and the second when her partner was drinking heavily. Both of these admissions were at her own request and were precipitated by increasing thoughts of self-harm, resulting in overdose.

Miss Jordash refused permission to interview her partner or to see her son. When asked she said, 'It's nothing to do with them, it's my problem.' She also refused to discuss any further the 'dirty episode' during her childhood, saying that she couldn't remember it clearly and she didn't want to develop 'false memory syndrome through questioning', which she had seen on the television. She did clarify that 'it' only happened once and, when asked directly, she said it had not involved any sexual abuse.

Miss Jordash attended the outpatient department on a weekly basis for two months and then fortnightly. She decided that she did not want to go to a residential unit and be separated from her son. However, she agreed to being referred to the local psychotherapy unit, where she was assessed and offered treatment. Since the waiting list for this was about one year she continued to attend the outpatient department on a regular basis.

## Reassessment

### Diagnosis

All the information obtained supports the diagnosis of an emotionally unstable personality disorder of borderline type. She also has recurrent depressive episodes, which are currently in remission, and in the past she has suffered from an eating disorder, probably anorexia nervosa.

### Aetiology

Apart from the details of her previous contact with mental health services there is no additional, independent, information about her background, apart from what she has already revealed.

### Further information

If she develops sufficient trust in her psychiatrist she should continue to be encouraged to allow other informants to be interviewed.

### Management

The relationship with a therapist will often reflect the complexities experienced in other relationships. Therefore, even if Miss Jordash sees her therapist in a positive light, she is likely to alternate between idealization and intense negative feelings. In psychotherapy these emotions are considered 'transference' reactions and are an invaluable part of the therapeutic process. For this to work effectively, she will need to feel positively about her therapist from the beginning in order to develop sufficient trust. Only then will she feel safe enough to talk openly about her doubts in their relationship. Since her contact with her psychiatrist will be less intense it will be more difficult to contain this process in the outpatient department. However, even in this setting it should be anticipated that she would experience such feelings. The psychiatrist can help prepare her for subsequent therapy by maintaining a constant and reliable approach and by ensuring that the boundaries are maintained.

The antidepressant medication should continue indefinitely, since she has found it helpful and there is good evidence that it reduces the frequency and severity of relapse in individuals who are vulnerable to recurrent depression.

### Prognosis

In the short term Miss Jordash's prognosis is poor with regard to her personality difficulties, because these are ingrained and she seems to have little control over them. This needs to be balanced, however, against the fact that she has been able to modify her drinking habits in order to protect her son. Eventually, this will be determined by whether she is able to establish a sufficiently good relationship, initially with her psychiatrist and later with her therapist. The outlook for her depression is more positive, provided she continues her antidepressant medication indefinitely.

## Postscript

Over the following year she made significant strides in terms of reducing her episodes of self-harm. She attended her outpatient appointments regularly and on time, with only a few missed sessions. She felt more positive about herself and attributed this to both her psychiatrist and the support offered to her son by the local services. She also allowed her family to be seen and her partner to be interviewed, and accepted a recommendation that she, her partner and their son attend family therapy to help Connor with his behavioural difficulties. Eventually she saw a psychotherapist, but discontinued therapy after five sessions, because 'I did not get on with that woman'. She continued to see her psychiatrist on a regular basis.

*Chapter 14*

# A Poor Historian

## *Mr Stone*

### Presenting complaint

Mr Stone was referred to the psychiatric outpatient department by his general practitioner who, in his referral letter, described him as 'forgetful and confused'. He attended with his mother, but they arrived at 6 p.m. and had to be seen by the emergency psychiatrist. Mr Stone was unable to explain why he was sent along to the outpatient department and the following account was therefore obtained from his mother.

She said that he had become very depressed over the last eight months. He started visiting her every Sunday and spent the whole day staring at the floor, muttering and saying very little. He ate very little and had lost a considerable amount of weight over this period. She attributed these changes to his poor accommodation, which was deteriorating as a result of a leaking roof. However, she thought that his problems really began about three years before, when his wife was divorcing him.

### Family history

Mr Stone's father was a frequent gambler and heavy drinker. He often beat his wife and when Mr Stone was about five years old she left him. Afterwards, his father suffered a 'nervous breakdown' and was admitted to a psychiatric hospital. He had no further contact with anyone in his family. Mrs Stone remarried three years later and she described her second husband as a 'very warm-hearted, kind man', who seemed to get on well with her family. He died suddenly of a stroke when Mr Stone was 18 years old.

Mr Stone's mother was 86 years old and presented herself as a capable, industrious woman. She continued to work as a cloth-cutter until her late 60s. During her retirement she remained fully independent and maintained close contact with all her children, whom she saw frequently. In spite of her relative fitness and her concern about her son's welfare, she said that she thought that she would be unable to take full responsibility for looking after him because of her increasing age and because he was becoming 'such a handful'.

Mr Stone had two older sisters. Mavis was 63 and a widow. She had been a successful student and matriculated at school. Two years previously she retired from managing a grocery store. June was 58 and single; she continued to work part time as a fabric buyer and lived with Mavis. The whole family lived within walking distance and maintained close and regular contact with each other.

## Personal history

Mr Stone's birth and early development were normal. He attended school until the age of 14 and was considered an average student. While there he involved himself in numerous sporting activities and made plenty of friends. When he left school he was initially apprenticed to a plumber, but two years later he became a carpenter's mate. In 1943, when he was 18, he was conscripted into the Royal Navy. Although he never saw active service, he spent eight months patrolling the North Sea in a motor torpedo boat. There was an occasion when he and some friends went absent without leave, as a result of which he spent three weeks in jail. He was never promoted and was demobbed in 1947, when he was 22 years old. Afterwards he had a variety of jobs, the longest of these lasted for 12 years, as a van driver. For the past five years he had worked part time in an amusement arcade and, as far as his mother was aware, he had continued this on a fairly regular basis until his presentation to the hospital.

When he was 18 he married a girl he had known for six months, but this never developed into a stable relationship and his wife had several affairs while he was in the Navy. This marriage ended in divorce when he was 23. During the next eight years he had several girlfriends, but never lived with, or became engaged to, any of them. When he was 32 he married a 35-year-old Spanish woman whom he met while she was working as a waitress in London. She was a single parent with an 18-year-old daughter who lived in Spain. Mr Stone's mother always thought of her as the dominant partner in their relationship and often referred to her during the interview as a 'nagger'. The couple had twins within a year of marriage and one son suffered a respiratory arrest when he was one year old, following an episode of pneumonia. He developed a learning disability, was statemented as having special educational needs and was sent to remedial classes at school, but was never institutionalized.

Mrs Stone had decided to return to work when the twins were two years old, and Mr Stone's mother looked after them until they reached the age of eleven. During this time the marriage steadily deteriorated. Mr and Mrs Stone had frequent rows about their son's welfare, her claims to independence and the extent to which she felt that his mother was attempting to organize their lives for them. These arguments became increasingly acrimonious and Mrs Stone continually accused him of 'turning out like his father'. They eventually separated and Mrs Stone took over complete responsibility for the twins' care when they were 11 years old. Their daughter did well at school and passed three GCE A levels, and their son moved from school to a community day centre. Following their separation Mr and Mrs Stone's relationship deteriorated further and she divorced him three years before his referral to hospital. Since then he had no further contact with either his wife or his children and, as far as Mr Stone's mother was aware, he had not acquired a new girlfriend.

Mr Stone had not generally been a regular or heavy drinker, but during the period surrounding his separation from his wife he frequently became drunk and abused her, both physically and verbally. His mother knew few details of this episode but believed that it never led to any contact with the police. As far as she knew he drank very little alcohol at the present time.

## Past medical history

Mr Stone received medical treatment for a perforated duodenal ulcer three years after he separated from his wife. He also suffered from a severe attack of 'bronchitis and asthma' which required inpatient treatment a year later. Apart from these illnesses he had been physically fit all his life. He was taking no prescribed medication and was a non-smoker.

## Past psychiatric history

Mr Stone had never previously seen a psychiatrist.

## Previous personality

His mother said that he was always an easy-going, sociable person and that he had many friends who frequently sought his company.

## Mental state examination

### Appearance and general behaviour

Mr Stone was a tall, thin, handsome man who sat hunched up in his chair, staring at his feet. He made few gestures, apart from intermittently taking his reading glasses out of their case, putting them on, taking them off and then returning them to their case. He was casually but tidily dressed, appeared clean but had a noticeable growth of stubble on his chin.

### Speech

Mr Stone said nothing except in response to direct questions, when he would nod and say a few words before trailing off into mumble. For example, when he was asked if he had any problems he said, 'I start to do something and…' When he was prompted he said, 'Well, um…' When he did speak it was quietly and at a normal rate.

### Mood

He looked miserable and his eyes frequently moistened, although he never actually cried. Occasionally he smiled in response to the interviewer's efforts to encourage him to speak.

*Thought content*

It was impossible to find out what Mr Stone was thinking because of his limited responses.

*Abnormal beliefs and interpretations of events*

None were elicited.

*Abnormal experiences*

None were elicited.

*Cognitive state*

Mr Stone knew the place and the year. However, he was unable to be more specific than this, despite prompting. When he was asked the date of the last war he replied, 'I can't remember dates.' He was then asked to subtract seven from 100, but remained silent.

*Self-appraisal*

This could not be elicited.

## Physical examination

A brief physical examination was carried out, which revealed no obvious abnormality except for evidence of weight loss.

## Preliminary assessment

Mr Stone is a middle-aged man who was brought to the psychiatric department by his mother. Over the last eight months he has become increasingly isolated, his mood has changed and he has lost a considerable amount of weight. His behaviour has deteriorated over the last few years, following his divorce, and this was associated with episodes of physical illness and heavy drinking. On examination he was miserable and showed poor concentration and memory. However, the most marked abnormality was his inability to initiate or maintain a conversation.

The unusualness of Mr Stone's presentation is worrying. The assessment needs to focus on the immediate management plans, which will include the possibility of hospitalization and the organization of special investigations.

## Diagnosis

The changes described in Mr Stone, in the presence of his disturbed mood and cognition, could be caused either by depression or by a dementing illness. The information available is insufficient to make a clear distinction between these, although depression would be a far more likely diagnosis than dementia in a 55-year-old man. However, there are certain features in Mr Stone's case that make dementia more likely. Although he seems miserable, he does not demonstrate the severe manifestations of depression that would explain his near muteness. In particular, this appears to be a manifestation of his poverty of thought rather than a reflection of depressive retardation.

## Aetiology

At this stage the relevance of aetiological factors to Mr Stone's condition depends upon whether they point towards a particular diagnosis or suggest fruitful lines of enquiry that might help clarify the diagnosis. For example, there is the possibility of an hereditary component since Mr Stone's father was also admitted to a psychiatric hospital. However, unless his father's diagnosis can be discovered this information is not helpful. As far as the possibility of depression is concerned, Mr Stone's past history provides conflicting evidence about his vulnerability to psychiatric disorder. He seems to have had considerable difficulties in establishing and maintaining long-term relationships with women and his separation from his second wife was associated with severe alcohol abuse and violent behaviour. These changes could be seen as a 'depressive equivalent' and would be consistent with his mother's suggestion that the final divorce from his wife had triggered off a 'depression'. On the other hand he has suffered from other severe stresses in his life – imprisonment for being absent without leave, a previous divorce, having a severely handicapped son – without any serious psychological complications.

If Mr Stone turns out to have a dementing illness it will be essential to consider all possible reversible causes, however unlikely these may be. These can be divided into the following: metabolic (myxoedema, hypercalcaemia, vitamin B12 and folic acid deficiency, and liver disease); infective (syphilis or a cerebral abscess); traumatic (especially a chronic sub-dural haematoma, which might follow a relatively trivial head injury); and finally, neoplastic, either primary or secondary. Mr Stone's history of drinking raises the suspicion of liver disease and his marked weight loss might have been associated with an underlying medical disorder. The other major causes of dementia are degenerative and cerebrovascular. Mr Stone's history of gradual deterioration without any step-wise episodes is more consistent with a parenchymal disorder such as Alzheimer's disease, which frequently occurs in this age group.

*Further information*

The major aim at this stage is to clarify the diagnosis. The most important aspect of this will therefore be a more detailed examination of Mr Stone's mental state, in particular an appraisal of his mood and cognitive functions. In addition to finding out whether Mr Stone has any depressive preoccupations, observations will need to be made of any variation in his mood, alteration in his sleep pattern or general evidence of retardation. He will also need a full and detailed examination of his cognitive skills, which includes tests of memory, orientation and concentration. An assessment of specific topographical cerebral functions should also be undertaken.

If it becomes clearer that Mr Stone is suffering from a depressive illness it will be necessary to obtain more detail about its mode of onset and its relationship to his separation from his wife. However, should it become clearer that Mr Stone's illness is organic in nature then it will be important to find out whether he has suffered from any head injury, however trivial. In either case a detailed account of his drinking habits will need to be obtained.

Mr Stone presents one of those clinical situations in which a physical examination is imperative. Particular attention will have to be paid to any evidence of liver, cardiovascular or neurological disease, each of which might be associated with a dementing illness. A bronchopulmonary neoplasm can also produce 'non-metastatic' effects similar to those found in Mr Stone and therefore needs to be excluded.

Special investigations are also required when investigating the possibility of a dementing illness. These are important not only to help reach a diagnosis, but also to exclude possible reversible causes of dementia. The routine investigations should include:

- full blood picture, serum B12 and serum folic acid
- blood urea and electrolytes, liver function tests and thyroid function tests, serum calcium
- VDRL (specific tests for syphilis)
- chest X-ray and electrocardiogram
- electroencephalogram (EEG), MRI or CT scan.

## Management

Mr Stone should be admitted to hospital immediately because of the significant deterioration that has taken place in his level of function and the uncertainty surrounding his diagnosis. If he is found to have a depressive illness it will require urgent treatment. Furthermore, as an inpatient, it will be easier to undertake the essential investigations which include detailed nursing observations of his behaviour and an assessment of his functional capacity.

## Prognosis

This depends upon the diagnosis that is eventually made. If Mr Stone is found to be suffering from depression then this should respond well to appropriate treatment. However, if the diagnosis is a dementing illness then the outcome is poor, unless a reversible primary cause can be found.

## Further details

Mr Stone was admitted to the ward. No further information was obtained from his mother about his recent deterioration and his ex-wife was not contacted. His mother insisted that he had only drunk heavily at the time of his separation from his ex-wife and confirmed that his deterioration had been a gradual one, with no sudden changes.

The nurses reported that he always looked miserable although he did seem more cheerful when his relatives visited. He slept well, attended regularly for meals, and ate all the food that was placed in front of him. He never spoke to other patients and ward staff unless they approached him and tended to remain isolated. On several occasions he left the ward, but he always returned before suppertime. He dressed and undressed himself and knew how to find his own bed and the toilet. He was never incontinent.

## Cognitive examination (performed one week after admission)

Mr Stone remained a rather dishevelled looking man. When interviewed he sat quite still and looked uncomfortable with a puzzled look on his face. He followed simple requests such as to take off his jacket, or to undo his buttons.

*General knowledge.* When he was asked to name the Prime Minister Mr Stone gave the name of the leader of the opposition. He knew the Queen's name, but when asked the name of her husband he replied, 'I don't know.' He remained silent or replied 'I don't know' when asked other questions about general events in the news.

*Orientation.* He knew the name of the town he lived in, but was only able to say he was in hospital after being prompted by being offered several alternatives: 'hospital, railway station, post office'. He named the year correctly, but replied 'I don't know' when asked to name the day and the month. When asked what time it was he replied 'after lunch' when it was 4 p.m. When he was asked to give his address, he remembered the name of the road, but said 'I can't remember' when asked the number of his house. He eventually gave the correct number when he was offered three alternatives.

*Past memory.* He remembered his year of birth, but was unable to state the day and month in spite of prompting. When he was asked his age he replied '45' and repeated this. He correctly gave the age when he had joined the Royal Navy, but when asked how old he was when he had left he said, 'The 1940s.' On repeating this question he replied, 'I don't know.'

*Recent memory.* He was able to repeat immediately the examining doctor's name, 'Dr Williams.' However, five minutes later he replied, 'Mr Wilson.' When he was asked to repeat 'Mr Albert Smith, 24, Peace Road, Southampton', his immediate reply was, 'Mr Albert...' Five minutes later he was unable to remember that he had been asked to remember an address.

*Concentration.* He counted up to 19 and stopped when requested to do so. He was then asked to subtract seven from 100 and replied 'one hundred'. In spite of further prompting he was unable to get beyond this.

*Simple arithmetic.* When he was asked to add seven and four he said, 'I don't know' and in spite of prompting did not give an answer.

*Object naming.* He was able to name correctly 'glasses' and 'buckle'. However, he called a watch 'a digit', a watchstrap 'a hand', an ashtray 'to put cigarettes in' and a jacket 'a cloak'.

*Picture copying and construction.* Mr Stone was asked to copy several shapes and to fill in the numbers on a clock face drawn by the doctor; he performed very poorly on these tasks and the clock showed 'crowding'.

## Physical examination

A thorough general examination was normal, apart from evidence of weight loss. In particular, his blood pressure was 120/80, there were no carotid or cardiac bruits and there was no clinical evidence to suggest that he had a neoplasm. The following features were noted in his nervous system. He was right-handed and showed no evidence of right/left disorientation. He was able to take his jacket off and put it on again correctly. No abnormalities were found in his visual fields or his cranial nerves. Examination of his motor and sensory systems and of his reflexes was normal. No primitive reflexes (sucking, grasping) were elicited. There was no evidence that he ignored any parts of his body (anosognosia) and he showed no manifestations of astereognosis, agraphaesthesia, sensory extinction or visual inattention. Cerebellar functions were also normal. All the special investigations were within normal limits, apart from the EEG and MRI scan.

## EEG

'A bilateral abnormality is noted. The dominant frequency is slow and there is rhythmic theta activity over the frontal region. This latter feature is more evident on the left, but there are no focal features.'

## MRI head scan

'Moderately severe, widespread atrophic changes. No focal lesions are seen.'

## Reassessment

### Diagnosis

The more detailed examination of Mr Stone's mental state confirms the severe impairment of his cognitive functions. He is more disorientated in time than in space, he also has a very poor grasp of general knowledge and a poor memory for past events, and he shows extremely distorted retention of recent events. His concentration is disturbed and he has acalculia. He also demonstrates nominal dysphasia, severe visuospatial agnosia and dysgraphia, and his drawing of a clock face showed marked 'crowding'.

He continues to show poverty of speech and although he is miserable, there is a shallowness about his mood that conveys a sense of perplexity. These features are consistent with generalized cortical disturbance, particularly loss of parietal lobe function. The EEG has confirmed the generalized nature of this dysfunction and his MRI scan also shows signs of widespread cortical atrophy. These features are all consistent with a diagnosis of dementia of the Alzheimer type, which must be the most likely diagnosis, given the absence of any other primary cause. In particular, his mother confirmed that there had been no step-wise deterioration, which would have suggested a diagnosis of arteriosclerotic dementia and there was no evidence of extrapyramidal symptoms, visual hallucinations or fluctuating levels of consciousness, which may suggest Lewy body dementia.

The possibility that Mr Stone's deterioration is secondary to an affective illness now seems very unlikely. No serious manifestation of depression has been observed by the nursing or medical staff and although he appears miserable this is conveyed in a rather shallow fashion. The fact that he seems perplexed is also consistent with a diagnosis of dementia. Although it remains possible that Mr Stone has a mild, coexisting affective disorder, this is unlikely to have contributed significantly to his symptom, which all point to a serious organic deficit.

### Aetiology

No new factors have emerged, although it is known that there may be a hereditary component to Alzheimer's dementia.

### Further information

It is now important to establish the level of independent function that Mr Stone will be able to sustain. A detailed occupational therapy report needs to be obtained, which should include an assessment of his ability to look after himself independently in his own home. He might be able to continue living independently with support from his family and back-up from the social services, including meals-on-wheels and visits from a community psychiatric nurse.

In view of the reported leaking roof a thorough evaluation should be made of the quality of his accommodation and its suitability for someone in his condition. At this stage it would also be useful to find out what Mr Stone does when he leaves the hospital.

### Management

The main aim of management is to support Mr Stone in the community as long as possible. Further assessments should be obtained as quickly as possible and appropriate social service support should be mobilized rapidly. This is likely to include a home help, meals-on-wheels, a community psychiatric nurse and attendance at a day centre. Arrangements will also need to be made to maintain contact with him in the outpatient department. If he is capable of living independently admission to a warden-controlled flat or an old age home may be necessary. At some time he may require admission to a care of the elderly ward, as his condition is almost certain to deteriorate.

Acetylcholinesterase inhibitors have been demonstrated to improve functioning in mild to moderate Alzheimer's dementia. This will require a specialist assessment.

It will be essential to keep Mr Stone's general practitioner fully informed of these details. His family should also be informed of the diagnosis and of its implications and will need to be consulted regarding the most appropriate way of providing support.

*Prognosis*

Alzheimer's disease has a poor long-term prognosis and 50 per cent of patients die within five years of the diagnosis being made. Features suggesting a worse outlook include an early age of onset, parietal lobe signs and rapid deterioration. In the short term the outlook may depend upon the presence of complicating factors such as depression. He is functioning surprisingly well, considering the severity of his deficits. For example, he orientated himself well in the ward following his admission to hospital. He also has no features of depression. On the other hand his illness began when he was quite young and he seems to have deteriorated quite significantly over the last year. In the long term, his prognosis is inevitably poor.

## Postscript

Mr Stone was referred to the local old age psychiatrist for assessment. It was decided that he did not meet criteria for medical treatment because his cognitive impairment was too severe. However, he was admitted for a subsequent trial of a novel acetylcholinesterase inhibitor, but this had no impact on his cognition or level of functioning.

He was also given a course of SSRIs in order to see whether this would lead to any improvement in his mental state. Following a two-month trial at a therapeutic dosage, no change was observed.

No functional assessment was made of Mr Stone. Since it was thought, on clinical grounds, he would be unable to maintain himself in the community he and his family were advised that he should apply for residential care. His family were unhappy about this and there was a considerable delay in arranging for an appropriate assessment. Three months after his admission a nurse reported that she had seen him going into an amusement arcade, one mile away from the hospital, every day. This turned out to be his previous place of employment, and he was spending the whole day there sitting in a corner. Following this discovery it was decided to try and support him at home and, after discussion with his family, he was encouraged to spend several weekends at home, all of which passed without mishap. One month later he was discharged home and arrangements were made for outpatient attendance and regular support. His family were advised to contact their local social services should the situation deteriorate. Six months later Mr Stone failed to attend any of the outpatient appointments made for him and his social worker was unable to contact either him or his family.

# Index